Contents

List of figures

The Care Process

Assessment, Planning, Implementation and
Evaluation in Health and Social Care

Health and Social Care titles from Reflect Press Ltd

Clinical Skills for Student Nurses edited by Robin Richardson
ISBN 978 1 906052 04 1
Understanding Research and Evidence-based Practice by Bruce Lindsay
ISBN 978 1 906052 01 0
Values for Care Practice by Sue Cuthbert and Jan Quallington
ISBN 978 1 906052 05 8
Communication and Interpersonal Skills by Elaine Donnelly and
Lindsey Neville
ISBN 978 1 906052 06 5
Numeracy, Clinical Calculations and Basic Statistics by Neil Davison
ISBN 978 1 906052 07 2
Essential Study Skills edited by Marjorie Lloyd and Peggy Murphy
ISBN 978 1 906052 14 0
Safe and Clean Care by Tina Tilmouth with Simon Tilmouth
ISBN 978 1 906052 08 9
Neonatal Care edited by Amanda Williamson and Kenda Crozier
ISBN 978 1 906052 09 6
Fundamentals of Diagnostic Imaging edited by Anne-Marie Dixon
ISBN 978 1 906052 10 2
Fundamentals of Nursing Care by Anne Llewellyn and Sally Hayes
ISBN 978 1 906052 13 3
The Care and Wellbeing of Older People edited by Angela Kydd, Tim Duffy
and F.J. Raymond Duffy
ISBN 978 1 906052 15 7
Palliative Care edited by Elaine Stevens and Janette Edwards
ISBN 978 1 906052 16 4
Nursing in the UK: A Handbook for Nurses from Overseas
by Wendy Benbow and Gill Jordan
ISBN 978 1 906052 00 3
Interpersonal Skills for the People Professions edited by Lindsey Neville
ISBN 978 1 906052 18 8
Understanding and Helping People in Crisis by Elaine Donnelly, Briony Williams and
Tess Parkinson
ISBN 978 1 906052 21 8
A Handbook for Student Nurses by Wendy Benbow and Gill Jordan
ISBN 978 1 906052 19 5
Professional Practice in Public Health edited by Jill Stewart and Yvonne Cornish
ISBN 978 1 906052 20 1

For further details on these and other Reflect Press titles please visit our
main website at **www.reflectpress.co.uk**

For Ebooks and free online resources please visit:
www.reflectpress-success.co.uk – the website supporting study success for health and
social care students.

The Care Process

Assessment, Planning, Implementation and Evaluation in Health and Social Care

Sally Hayes and Anne Llewellyn

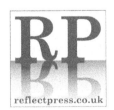

Reflect Press Ltd
www.reflectpress.co.uk
www.reflectpress-success.co.uk

First published in 2010

ISBN: 978 1 906052 22 5

British Library Cataloguing in Publication Data
A catalogue record for this book is available from the British Library

Production project management by Deer Park Productions
Typeset by Kestrel Data, Exeter, Devon
Cover design by Design Intoto
Printed and bound by Bell & Bain Ltd, Glasgow
Distributed by BEBC, Albion Close, Parkstone, Poole, Dorset BH12 3LL

Published by Reflect Press Ltd
11 Attwyll Avenue
Exeter
Devon, EX2 5HN
UK
01392 204400
www.reflectpress.co.uk
www.reflectpress-success.co.uk

List of tables

List of abbreviations

ACE – Angiotensin Converting Enzyme

ASPIRE – acronym for Assessment, Planning, Implementation, Review and Evaluation of Care

CFP – Common Foundation Programme (Nursing)

CHRE – Council for Health Care Regulation Excellence

CPA – Care Programme Approach

CAF – Common Assessment Framework

CQC – Care Quality Commission

CSCI – Commission for Social Care Inspectorate

CVA – Cerebral Vascular Accident

CWDC – Children's Workforce Development Council

DASS – Director of Adult Social Services

DFEE – Department for Education and Employment

DH – Department of Health

DHSS – Department of Health and Social Services

EBP – Evidence-based Practice

ESC – Essential Skills Clusters

FACS – Fair Access to Care Services

GDP – Gross Domestic Product

GP – General Practitioner

GSCC – General Social Care Council

JRF – Joseph Rowntree Foundation

JRHT – Joseph Rowntree Housing Trust

LA – Local Authority

LINks – Local Involvement Networks

LTCs – Long-Term Conditions

MACROS – Measurable, Achievable and time-limited, Client-centred, Realistic, Outcome written and Short

MHPIG – Mental Health Policy Implementation Guide

MHRA – Medicines and Healthcare products Regulatory Agency

MCA – Mental Capacity Act

MDT – Multi-disciplinary Team

MP – Member of Parliament

MS – Multiple Sclerosis
NCIL – National Centre for Independent Living
n.d. – no date
NG Tube – Naso-gastric Tube
NHS – National Health Service
NHSCCA – National Health Service and Community Care Act
NICE – National Institute for Health and Clinical Excellence
NMC – Nursing and Midwifery Council
NOS – National Occupational Standards
NSF – National Service Framework
ONS – Office for National Statistics
PAF – Performance Assessment Framework
PALS – Patient Advisory Liaison Service
Para – Paragraph
PbR – Payment by Results
PCT – Primary Care Trust
PEST – Political, Economic, Social, Technological
PI – Performance Indicator
PROMs – Patient Reported Outcome Measures
QAA – Quality Assurance Agency
QALYs – Quality Adjusted Life Years
REEPIG – Realistic, Explicit, Evidence-based, Prioritised, Involved and Goal-centred
SCIE – Social Care Institute for Excellence
SAP – Single Assessment Process
SFC – Skills for Care
SMART – Specific, Measurable, Achievable, Realistic, Timely
SOLER – Sit, Open, Lean, Eye, Relax (Communication Model)
SS – Social Services
SSD – Social Service Department
TOPSS – Training Organisation for Personal Social Services
UK – United Kingdom
UKCC – United Kingdom Central Council (Preceded NMC)
WHO – World Health Organisation
WWII – World War Two

Acknowledgements

We would like to thank our respective families and friends for their support and forbearance while we have been writing this book, with particular thanks to Anne Moseley for her continuous support and encouragement. We are very grateful to Nick Frost and Judith Harvey for their helpful comments and constructive feedback on the earlier drafts of the book.

Introduction

In our book entitled *The Fundamentals of Nursing Care: A Textbook for Students of Nursing and Health Care* (2008) we explored the concept of 'caring', emphasising the importance of patient-centred and patient-led care, and the importance of ensuring quality and using holistic principles. The humanistic aspects of nursing care, which are highly valued by the recipients of care (DH, 2002a), were explored, defined and, where possible, quantified in order that students of health care disciplines could examine and reflect on them in order to enable them to not only value these aspects of care delivery, but also understand their impact and relevance within the therapeutic encounter.

Another key element of professional care and practice is the need for accurate and robust processes of care, so that individual service user and carer needs are met in a personalised and comprehensively planned manner. This is becoming increasingly important due to changing demographics in the UK, with more people living longer with increasingly complex health and social care needs. This also means that inter-agency working, which can be complicated and at times challenging to orchestrate, is imperative.

ASPIRE

One way of conceptualising this care process is demonstrated by Sutton (1999) who uses the acronym ASPIRE to identify the different elements within the care process:

- ASsessment;
- Planning;
- Implementation;
- Review and Evaluation.

This process is cyclical and continuous, as review and evaluation may lead on to further assessment, starting the process again as assessment is ongoing and not a one-off activity. It is a process in which needs are continuously assessed and re-assessed according to ongoing evaluation.

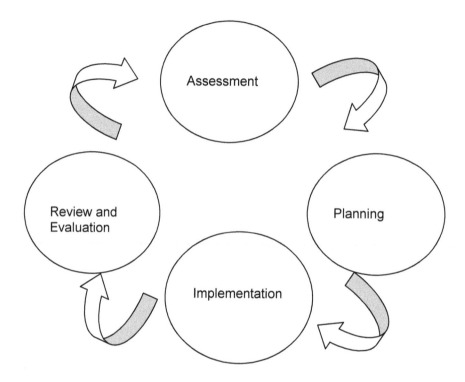

Figure 1 Diagrammatic representation of the cyclical process of care

Throughout many areas of decision-making in our lives, we may adopt this cyclical approach to decision-making and activities. Imagine, for example, someone is planning a party. The organiser will need to follow a process, which includes the need to assess, plan, implement and evaluate. In the assessment, the relevant factors may be:

- What is the purpose of the party?
- What sort of party will it be?
- Where will it be held?
- Who needs to be involved in the decision-making and organisation?

Fundamental to these questions will be the issues of finance and available resources. Planning will therefore involve matching the resources to the available options, planning the types of refreshments and entertainments that will be provided, and deciding who will be invited. All of these factors will depend on available budget and personal preferences.

Implementation will focus on the hosting of the party and, although there may not be a formal evaluation, consideration of how it went, what worked well and what did not will influence whether the organiser would hold a similar party in the future and whether they would recommend any elements of the party to a friend.

This is similar to the process of ASPIRE in health and social care, where a number of questions need to be addressed in order to undertake an assessment of need and to gather the information required to plan care and interventions. Essentially, health and social care practice involves problem-solving and identifying solutions to problems, whether the individual is admitted to hospital for a short planned operation, or receives time-limited care within the primary care sector, or they have longer-term health and social care needs. The care process involves a series of stages and good assessment is essential for the identification of the problem as well as setting goals and planning interventions. If we fail to assess properly, there is a risk of interventions being based on guesswork or chance or of a ritualised approach to the care process (Thompson and Thompson, 2008; Ford and Walsh, 1994).

PROFESSIONAL STANDARDS

The importance of this systematic and cyclical approach to care for health and social care practice is demonstrated in the professional requirements for proficiency in both nursing and social work practice.

Professional standards for nursing care

The Nursing and Midwifery Council (NMC) governs the progression to Nursing branch programmes and registration for professional practice. This body is charged with setting the standards for the assessment and establishment of professional competency and proficiency, and has set 17 standards for proficiency that nurses must prove that they have attained in order to practice legally as a qualified practitioner (NMC, 2004). The standards focus on the cyclical process of care delivery and, as such, require nurses to demonstrate competence in the assessment, planning and implementation of nursing care within ethical, legal and policy frameworks. The proficiencies are also related to *The Code: The Standards of Conduct, Performance and Ethics for Nurses and Midwives* (NMC, 2008).

In 2007, the NMC produced 'Essential Skill Clusters' for Pre-registration Nursing Programmes, which established standards of proficiency required for entry to branch programmes and for entry to the register, enabling them to practice as qualified practitioners. These clusters focus on the holistic needs of service users and identify a more specific achievement of learning outcomes in relation to:

- care, compassion and communication;
- organisational aspects of care;
- infection prevention and control;
- nutrition and fluid management;
- medicines management.

The Essential Skills Clusters (ESCs) for nursing state that nurses should: 'Deliver care that addresses both physical and emotional needs and preferences' (ESC 5) (NMC, 2007). Other clusters identify the centrality of assessment to specific features of care, such as nutrition (ESC 28) and infection control (ESC 21).

Professional standards for social work practice

The General Social Care Council is the body charged with setting the standards for social work practice and, in conjunction with the Department of Health (2002) and the Training Organisation for Personal Social Services (TOPSS), has established National Occupational Standards (NOS) for practice that social workers must achieve in order to progress through the levels of their course and be registered as a qualified practitioner. These occupational standards focus on a wide range of skills and competencies required for practice and reflect the subject benchmarks established by the Quality Assurance Agency (QAA). Assessment is a key competency for social work practice, as evidenced in National Occupational Standard 2:

- Assess needs properly: making sure that all options are explored before deciding on a plan (NOS 2h);
- Assess risk and support risk taking when appropriate (NOS 2j).

THE IMPORTANCE OF POLICY

Before we move on to the wider professional context and process of ASPIRE it is important to recognise the importance of the policy context. Policy is set by the Department of Health and essentially sets national strategy and overall direction for the NHS and Social Services (Pollock and Talbot-Smith, 2006). Policy is important to the ASPIRE process as it influences the work of health and social care practitioners at all levels. For example, policy impacts on diverse areas of practice from the amount of resources that are available to fund (or not fund) a service, to the types of practitioners that are legally enabled or 'legitimised' to undertake certain tasks and roles.

THE CONTENT, COVERAGE AND APPROACH OF THIS BOOK

It is within the professional and policy context that we will explore the process of delivering high quality, service user-led care in this book. The book is intended as a foundation level text, which focuses on fundamental principles of ASPIRE and the related context in health and social care. It is set out as a workbook, using case narratives to stimulate reflective learning and ground theoretical perspectives. The book can therefore be used as an independent study tool or as a core text within a particular module and, in pedagogical terms, it will promote:

- Enquiry-based learning or problem-based learning (Rideout, 2001), which is based around the concept that the starting point of learning should be a problem or a query that the individual student wishes to solve (Boud *et al.*, 1985);
- Critical thinking, which is a central tenet of reflective practice (Moon, 2004);
- The exposure of tacit knowledge through reflection which promotes self-awareness and enables practitioners to evaluate their practice (Jasper, 1999);
- The use of case studies as tools for reflective thinking, thus developing the ability of students to deconstruct practice and examine how to further develop competencies.

(Adapted from Llewellyn and Hayes, 2008)

Chapter 1 sets the scene by defining health and social care. This is important in terms of the care process as it will help you to understand the historical context of the development of health and social care as concerns of both the policy-makers and professionals. Definitions of health and health behaviours are explored and the historical development of health and social care are examined with reference to the biomedical and social models of health care. The chapter considers the importance of user and carer perspectives in health and social care delivery, exploring the concept of power within these relationships. This traces the origins of why the care process looks as it does by examining the role of the individuals and their specific roles as 'service user', 'carer' or 'professional practitioner'. The relationship between health and social care is also scrutinised, emphasising the importance of joint working between health and social care agencies in the provision of holistic person-centred care.

Chapter 2 considers the politics and key policy drivers in health and social care, defining policy and exploring the factors that influence policy and policy-making including:

- demographics;
- evidence-based practice;
- technological and pharmaceutical advances;
- the impact on health and social care of the rise in the incidence of Long-Term Conditions;
- globalisation;
- consumerism or the consumer culture.

Consideration is also given to the increasing focus on quality and the important issues about resources and finance. An understanding of the policy context is essential in understanding the care process as it dictates the very manner in which ASPIRE is undertaken through funding and the establishment of national, regional and local policy targets and standards.

Chapter 3 examines the contemporary context of health and social care practice by considering key contemporary issues including the transformation of adult social care services, health care modernisation, person-centred care, personalisation and self-directed support, and, importantly, risk and safeguarding. It examines and explains the impact of these issues on the care process by changing the focus of policy and thus standards.

Chapters 4 to 7 then explore the process of care by considering the four-stepped process of ASPIRE – Assessment, Planning, Implementation and Review and Evaluation.

Finally, Chapter 8 concludes the discussion with the consideration of future challenges for health and social care. It encourages health and social care practitioners to take an active and empowering (even emancipatory) approach to future health and social care delivery.

The book has been designed to support and extend students' learning, introducing key concepts in relation to the ASPIRE process. Case studies and structured activities are employed to engage the reader and help them to understand relevance to their health and social care practice. Each chapter has clearly defined learning outcomes and a short annotated bibliography to guide students to further reading. Relevant key social work roles from the National Occupational Standards for Social Work and key nursing skills from the Essential Skills Clusters will be identified throughout the book.

The case studies throughout the book are fictional, although some elements of them may be derived from real situations to ensure authenticity. The biographical data and details of locations are all fictional and any resemblance to reality is accidental and coincidental.

Author Biographies

Anne Llewellyn is a Senior Lecturer and Teacher Fellow in the Faculty of Health at Leeds Metropolitan University. She has 17 years of experience of teaching diverse groups of students in nursing, social work and social sciences in Higher Education Institutions. Within a broad context of contemporary policy and ideological imperatives in health and social care, the particular emphasis of her teaching is on the application of subject specific and social scientific theories to inform professional practice and the use of narratives and reflective learning approaches to facilitate this learning and application.

Sally Hayes is a Senior Lecturer in the Faculty of Health at Leeds Metropolitan University with experience of teaching students at different academic levels within nursing and healthcare related professions. Her portfolio is focused particularly around Primary Health Care Provision and includes Health Policy, Leadership and Management and the development of Practice Teachers. She is particularly interested in facilitating the development of practitioners who base their practice on a journey of lifelong learning through critical reflection.

Chapter 1

Defining Health and Social Care

This chapter covers the following key issues:

- definitions of health and health behaviours;
- the historical development of health and social care;
- the importance of user and carer perspectives in health and social care delivery;
- the importance of joint working between health and social care agencies in the provision of person-centred care.

By the end of this chapter you should be able to:

- explain what is meant by a biomedical approach to health care;
- explain the key elements of a social model of health care;
- identify power relationships in the delivery of health and social care and the impact of these relationships for service user care;
- engage with debates about the relationship between health and social care for personal wellbeing.

This chapter matches to the following National Occupational Standards and Essential Skills Clusters:

- ESC 2.iii Actively encourages patient/client to be involved in, and/or ensures that they are supported in their own care;
- ESC 3.i Take a person-centred approach to care;
- ESC 3.ii Demonstrates respect for diversity and individual patient/client preference, regardless of personal view;
- ESC 4.i Demonstrates an understanding of how culture, religion, spiritual beliefs, gender and sexuality impact on illness and disability;
- ESC 4.ii Respects people's rights.

- NOS 2.2 Work with individuals, families, carers, groups and communities to identify, gather, analyse and understand information;
- NOS 2.3 Work with individuals, families, groups and communities to enable them to analyse, identify, clarify and express their strengths, expectations and limitations.

INTRODUCTION

When examining the care process it is of vital importance to understand how health care and social care have developed historically, so we can understand how they are currently defined within society. This chapter is about understanding 'needs' – how people define their own health and wellbeing needs, how 'needs' have been defined and addressed in the past, and how this has changed and developed into the modern holistic understanding of needs. The very process of ASPIRE is defined by the contemporary definition of health and social care need.

Activity

Before reading the next section, think about what health means to you.

1. What makes you decide that you feel healthy?
2. What makes you decide that you are unhealthy?

DEFINING HEALTH

Although the terms 'health' and 'healthy' are widely used in common speech and in health and social care environments, these terms are rather complex and difficult to define. In 1990 the Health and Lifestyles survey was carried out by a multi-disciplinary group of researchers to explore lay people's perceptions and views about health (Blaxter, 1990). They identified a number of different subjective definitions of health, which incorporated medical, social and holistic elements.

Definition	Sample response
Health:	
as not ill	Someone I know who is very healthy is me, because I haven't been to a doctor yet.
despite disease	I am very healthy despite this arthritis.
as a reserve	Both parents are still alive at 90 so he belongs to healthy stock.
as 'the healthy life'	I call her healthy because she goes jogging and doesn't eat fried food.
as physical fitness	There's tone to my body, I feel fit.
as energy or vitality	Health is when I feel I can do anything.
as social relationships	You feel as though everyone is your friend, I enjoy life more, and can work, and help other people.
as function	She's 81 and she gets her work done quicker than me, and she does the garden.
as psychosocial wellbeing	Well I think health is when you feel happy.

Table 1 Lay definitions of health (source: Blaxter (1990) *Health and Lifestyles*, Chapter 2)

We can see from the Blaxter (1990) research that health is defined in many different ways. To explore these definitions of health and their theoretical bases, we can broadly divide the definitions of health into three sub-categories:

1. The biomedical definition (the absence of disease model of health);
2. Social models of health, which see health as a social phenomenon;
3. Holistic models, which view health as determined by psychosocial, biological, environmental and spiritual factors (considered in more detail at the end of this chapter).

The biomedical approach to health and illness

The absence of disease model of health and illness is based on the medical model of health care, which has dominated formal health care delivery in the western world since the eighteenth century. This medical model or biomedical model developed as part of a wider social process of scientific development, and replaced previous unscientific explanations of health and illness, which viewed ill health either as an imbalance with the natural world, a punishment from an external force or being (such as a supernatural being) or based on the miasmic theory, where illness was viewed as the result of bad smells (Webster, 2001). The biomedical model of illness is based on five assumptions.

1. **The mechanical metaphor of the body** – the body can be broken down into component parts, and these component parts can be isolated and the dysfunctions treated, similar to the analogy of car maintenance and repair.
2. **Mind-body dualism** – the mind and body are seen as separate from one another, and therefore do not have any influence on each other.
3. **The doctrine of specific aetiology** – or cause and symptoms. Specific causes can be identified and treated for each disease.
4. **The technological imperative** – the merits and benefits of technological interventions (either through surgical and other invasive procedures or through pharmacological prescriptions) are valued.
5. **Reductionism** – the model reduces individuals to a set of anatomical and physiological processes, with lesser emphasis on psychosocial and environmental processes.

As stated above, the biomedical model has dominated formal health care in the UK and other Western capitalist societies since the eighteenth century, and has been widely seen as the only valid and objective way to diagnose and treat illnesses and diseases (Nettleton, 2006). Within this model then, health is equated with absence of disease and needs are assessed in terms of those factors that need to be addressed to rid the individual of disease or illness. For example, an individual who has hypothermia needs to have their core body temperature increased slowly until it returns to normal parameters.

Social models of health

The biomedical model has been criticised as it fails to account for subjective experiences of health and wellness, which impact on people's lives as well as their interpretations of symptoms and engagement with formal health care. In particular, sociologists have been critical of the biological imperative of care within the biomedical model, which is not only based on questionable claims of effectiveness and validity (Illich, 1976), but also removes health and illness from the socio-environmental context within which it occurs.

In the 1960s, the discipline of medical sociology developed as a sub-discipline of sociology. Medical sociologists not only questioned the validity and objectivity of the medical model of health care, but also proposed a social model to explain health and illness. Social models generally have three characteristics.

1. Health and illness are produced within a social context, influencing how people interpret and experience health and illness.
2. Social variables are important determinants of health and illness. While the biomedical model sees health and illness as a natural process, the social model acknowledges that social factors influence the biological processes. Thus, social variables such as class, gender, ethnicity and geographical location all impact both on disease and illness causation. Using the example of hypothermia above, the individual would not only need to have their core body temperature increased, but there would also be a need to assess the social factors that may have contributed to hypothermia – for example, whether their house is adequately heated, whether they have sufficient income to use heating, whether they have sufficient warm clothing.
3. Health care is not objective, but decisions are made based on people's personal characteristics. For example, there are differences in the way that men and women are diagnosed and treated based on gender stereotypes (Payne, 2006).

Activity

Have a look at the following websites and identify social variables that impact on health and illness.

www.archive.official-documents.co.uk/document/doh/ih/ ih.htm

www.dh.gov.uk/en/Publicationsandstatistics/Publications/ PublicationsPolicyAndGuidance/DH_082378

Understanding the subjective interpretation of health and illness is important when assessing and planning care, as it may impact on issues such as assessment of the need for professional involvement, compliance with planned interventions (for example, drug regimes) and self-assessment of needs. These issues will be discussed further later on in this chapter.

The functionalist approach to health

The work of Talcott Parsons (1951) has been particularly influential in identifying the social as well as biological basis of illness (Annandale, 1998). Parsons was a functionalist sociologist, believing that society is made up not just of individuals and their actions, but also of a series of inter-dependent systems and structures. The smooth running of society is dependent on individuals and these systems operating in harmony to maintain the status quo. Thus functionalists are interested in the roles that people have and how these roles and responsibilities are managed for the collective good.

For functionalists, the inability to maintain roles and responsibilities is seen as deviant, in that it disrupts the equilibrium and smooth running of society. To address this, Parsons developed the sick role concept, arguing that if people were unable to fulfil roles and responsibilities, then they should be assigned a new role, the sick role, which would exempt them from their obligations. However, these exemptions were based on obligations on the part of the sick person to get better. Thus the sick role is based on the following exemptions and obligations.

1. Exemption from normal social responsibilities (for example, work and family roles).
2. Exemption from responsibility for own illness (i.e., the sick person cannot be expected to get better through their own free will).
3. The obligation to be motivated to get better.
4. The obligation to seek technically competent help.

Parsons sees the medical profession as the objective providers of technically competent help, so although he sees illness as a social phenomenon as well as a biological malfunction, he concurs with the dominance of the biomedical model within the formal system of health care, and assumes that there is a uni-modal relationship between patient and doctor, with the doctor holding power in terms of diagnosis, treatment and referral.

This notion of personal roles and responsibilities fits with Blaxter's (1990) definition of health as function, in that health is seen as the ability to perform daily activities of living. Many professional models of care have focused on helping people to manage their daily activities of living, either through adaptation or rehabilitation and have used these functions as the basis for their model of assessment. Roper, Logan and Tierney (2000) developed a model for nursing practice in 1980, based on 12 activities of living, which should be viewed on the independence-dependence continuum. These activities of living are:

- maintaining a safe environment;
- communication;
- breathing;
- eating and drinking;
- elimination;
- washing and dressing;
- controlling temperature;
- mobilisation;
- working and playing;
- expressing sexuality;
- sleeping;
- death and dying.

Within this model of care, nurses are guided to assess the patient's ability to perform functions and to plan and implement a package of care to address any deficits (these issues will be developed further in Chapters 4-7). Similarly, occupational therapists use a model of activities of daily living when working to optimise individual independence, and social workers use a systems approach when working with individuals and families (Thompson and Thompson, 2008). A similar model of care is used by multi-disciplinary groups when working with older people with long-term care needs (Forster *et al.*, 2009).

LAY PERSPECTIVES OF HEALTH

Theories of health are therefore important in informing professional models of working with service users. However, lay perspectives on health are also important, as they locate health and health and illness behaviours within the context of people's individual lives and help us to understand the subjective experience of health and illness. This is increasingly important as the ASPIRE process is concerned with needs as identified by the care recipient themselves, and as self-assessment of needs becomes more central to the process of care delivery (see Chapter 4).

An interviewee from Blaxter and Patterson's (1982) research defines health as follows:

> After I was sterilised I had a lot of cystitis, and backache because of the fibroids. Then when I had a hysterectomy I had bother wi' my waterworks because my bladder lived a life of its own and I had to have a repair . . . Healthwise I would say I'm OK. I did hurt my shoulder – I mean this is nothing to do with health but I actually now have a disability, I get a gratuity payment every six months . . . I wear a collar and take Vallium . . . then, just the headaches – but I'm not really off work a lot with it.
>
> (p. 29)

This is an interesting quote, as it demonstrates the complex processes by which people judge their health and illness. Although this lady has a number of objective symptoms and, according to the biomedical model of health, would be seen as having ill health, she sees herself as healthy because she is able to carry out her normal work role. Thus she has assessed her health on the basis of her ability to perform her normal roles, as identified above.

Social roles in lay definitions of health

Social roles are important in lay definitions of health as identified by Blaxter (1990). The notions of wellbeing and social relationships are important within lay conceptualisations of health and illness, and these social concepts form an important aspect of human existence and social involvement.

Activity

Think of the different roles that you have within your family or social network. What responsibilities to other people do you have in these roles?

The impact of health and illness on social relationships and roles is based on subjective assessment, as individuals locate health and illness within the context of their own lives and belief and value systems. This personal assessment of health is known as a lay health belief, based on social factors as opposed to the medical model of health, which is seen as a professional model of health belief, based on objective and measurable

Medical Model	Social Model
A state of health is a biological fact: it is immutable, real, independent.	A state of health is socially constructed: it is varied, uncertain, diverse.
Ill health is caused by biological calamities: • 'entrants' to the body (e.g. viruses, germs); • 'internal faults' (e.g. genes); • trauma.	Ill health is caused by social factors: • behind the biology lies society; • root causes are social causes.
Causes are identified by: • signs and symptoms; • the process of 'diagnosis'; • from medically established 'normality'.	Causes are identified through: • beliefs, which are varying, subjective, society- and community-based; • interpretation, built up through custom and social constraint.
Medical knowledge is exclusionary: • it is the job of the expert or specialist; • facts are accumulated and built upon; • alternative perspectives are invalid and inferior.	Knowledge is not exclusionary: • it has a historical, cultural and social context; • it is shaped by involved people.
Biomedicine is reductionist and disease-oriented, concerned with pathology.	The social model is holistic and concerned with context.

Table 2 Summary of the differences between the medical model and the social model of health care (Moon and Gillespie, 1995)

criteria. Lay health beliefs are determined by a complex set of social factors, and are individual and unique, as opposed to the universal assumptions about health within the medical model. Lay definitions of health are therefore located within social environments and contexts and are influenced by social factors, such as class, gender, ethnicity, location in social structures and own personal experiences. Family, for example, plays a large role in shaping early perceptions and beliefs about health and illness. Sociologists see the family as an important unit of primary socialisation, where behaviours and beliefs are shaped (see, for example,

Macionis and Plummer, 2005; Llewellyn *et al.*, 2008) and Graham (1984) argues that the family plays an important role in shaping health beliefs and behaviours. Peers, the education system, the mass media and the professional sector may also influence health beliefs and behaviours.

> **Activity**
>
> Think about your own definition of health. How has this been influenced by behaviours learned within your family?

SOCIAL NEEDS

Social needs are much more difficult to define than health needs and, as discussed above, it is difficult to separate health needs from social needs. As discussed earlier in relation to health, there is a subjective element to the identification of needs, and there may be little agreement between individuals as to what constitutes a need.

> **Activity**
>
> 1. List 10 needs.
> 2.
>   a) Is there a pattern or logic in the list of needs you have drawn up?
>   b) Do some needs come before others?
>   c) Are some needs more basic or fundamental?
>   d) Is your list culture-free?
>   e) Which of these needs would you define as health needs?
>   f) Which of these needs would you define as social needs?

Social needs can be defined in a number of ways:

- **Felt needs** – individuals are conscious of their needs (Bradshaw, 1972), which incorporates a subjective element of interpretation. For example, an individual may feel that they need to be referred for physiotherapy to help them to mobilise more freely.
- **Expressed needs** – these are needs that are publicised and as these needs are known about, they can become demands. For example, the

recent media stories identifying postcode lottery provision of anti-cancer drugs has demonstrated how, as drugs become available, there is an expectation that they should be accessible to all who might benefit from them.

- **Normative needs** – these are needs that are defined according to professional norms or standards, which involves the input of outside observers or experts. This model of addressing need has been historically employed within the personal social services, as welfare professionals have had responsibility for assessing needs and planning interventions.

- **Comparative needs** – these incorporate the concept of relative judgement, and can be seen in the context of eligibility criteria and Fair Access to Care Services (FACS) policies (DH, 2002h), which have been implemented in health and social care (see Chapter 2).

Activity

Read the following case study and make a list of Frank's health and social care needs.

Frank is a 74-year-old retired postmaster, who has lived on his own since Marjorie, his wife of 47 years, died from cancer two years ago. She had been diagnosed with breast cancer six months before her death and, after her initial surgery and radiotherapy, Frank cared for her at home. Although both Frank and his wife wanted her to have a peaceful death at home, this was not possible as she was admitted to hospital as an urgent admission with complications just prior to her death.

Frank was diagnosed with Type II diabetes six years ago, and has been managing his diabetes through control of his diet, following consultation with the dietitian at the local health centre. Frank also has essential hypertension, which is controlled with 10 mg daily of the angiotensin converting enzyme (ACE) inhibitor, Ramipril.

Although Frank lives on his own, he has a married daughter who lives in the village five miles away, and he has regular contact with his daughter, son-in-law and three grandchildren. He also has a married son, who lives with his wife and two children some distance away, but maintains regular phone contact, and Frank goes to stay with the family at least twice a year. Frank enjoys his garden and takes pride in maintaining his extensive range of plants and flowers, as well as growing his own produce in his greenhouse and vegetable garden. He and his wife were members of the local church and Frank often supplied flowers from his garden for church displays. He has a wide circle of friends through his British Legion club who he meets with regularly.

Over the last few weeks Frank has been feeling very lethargic and tired and, although generally he has managed to cook for himself, he has become increasingly reliant on ready meals and take-away food. When his daughter visits, she notices that Franks looks tired and he is unkempt and withdrawn. The garden is overgrown and when she asks Frank about the British Legion, he tells her that he has not been for a few weeks. His daughter is worried that the house seems cold and in a poor state of repair. When she asks Frank about this, he says that he worries about the cost of heating the house. She is further concerned when she tests the smoke alarm and finds that it is not working.

See Appendix 2 for an example of a nursing care plan that outlines Frank's needs. See Appendix 3 for an example of a social care plan that outlines Frank's needs.

This case study demonstrates the complexity of the concept of need and the overlap between health needs and social care needs. Parry-Jones and Soulsby (2001) discuss the problems of assessing need, where there is a lack of conceptual clarity about the concept of need, and conclude that it is essential to clarify when something is a health need or social need if health and social care agencies are to effectively carry out their functions and work collaboratively to address the service user's needs. These issues will be discussed further and we will return to the case study about Frank at points throughout the book to demonstrate the ASPIRE process in practice.

THE COMPLEXITY OF HEALTH BELIEF SYSTEMS

It is increasingly acknowledged that there is an artificial distinction between the physical, social, professional and lay perspectives of health and decisions about health and social needs. Assessment of health and decisions about seeking health care are based on a complex set of belief systems and value judgements, incorporating social as well as biological factors. The ability to function both physically and socially is an important determinant of health. Ill health has biological and psychosocial consequences for the individual, and therefore needs to be seen within a social as well as a medical context. In addition, the social context is important in terms of illness behaviour. Although the historical development of formal health care has been dominated by the medical model of health and illness, much health care takes place within the popular sector of health care, which is dominated by lay expertise in health and illness.

Kleinman (1988) identifies three overlapping systems of health care that individuals access when experiencing ill health, the formal or professional sector, the informal or popular sector and the folk sector.

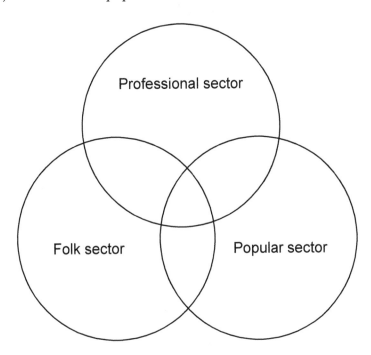

Figure 2 A diagrammatic representation of a model of health care (adapted from Kleinman, 1988)

The professional sector comprises the professions and institutions that make up the formal health care sector, such as hospitals, primary health care services, community care services, doctors, nurses and other health and social care practitioners. The folk sector is the part of health care that involves alternative and complementary care, while the popular sector is comprised of individuals, families, community networks and social networks. Within this model, the professional sector (based on the biomedical model of health care) is dominant in terms of power, but the popular sector is dominant in terms of its influence over health behaviours and illness decisions. Dingwall (1976) refers to the lay referral network in health care, where decisions about health and illness are determined within the popular sector of health care. This is especially important when individuals are making assessments about severity of symptoms and decisions to seek medical help (White, 2002). This demonstrates the fact that it is very difficult to separate the biomedical and social aspects of health and health care, as they influence each other. Mechanic (1962) illustrates this in his discussion of trigger factors that influence people's decisions to seek health care services within the formal sector of health care. Although formal health care and the biomedical model have dominance in terms of the legitimation of illness and treatment decisions, much health care takes place within the informal sector, and decisions to seek technically competent care are based on a complex set of health and social factors.

Trigger factors for seeking help in the formal sector of health care

The trigger factors for seeking help in the formal sector of health care have been identified as follows:

- visibility, recognisability or perceptual salience of symptoms;
- perceived seriousness of symptoms;
- extent to which symptoms disrupt family, work and other social activities;
- frequency of appearance of symptoms;
- tolerance thresholds;
- available knowledge, information and cultural assumptions;
- perceptual needs;
- needs competing with illness responses;
- competing possible interpretations that can be assigned to symptoms;
- availability of treatment resources.

(Mechanic, 1962)

These trigger factors are especially important as individuals make assessments about the severity of their symptoms and whether to seek medical help.

Activity

Think about the last time that you sought medical help.

1. What influenced your decision?
2. Can you identify who was involved in the assessment of your health and illness needs?

Power and control

Power and control are also important elements in understanding health and social care. Historically, health and social care has been dominated by the medical approach to health and illness, reflecting the power that the medical profession has. As stated above, health care has been dominated by the biomedical model and this was formalised in the UK with the introduction of the National Health Service in 1948, following the 1946 National Health Act (Klein, 2005).

THE HISTORICAL CONTEXT

Having examined the social and medical models of health and lay perspectives it is important to examine more broadly the historical context of health and social care as this helps to reveal how 'need' has been understood and interpreted in health and social care at different times by society. This in turn influences how need has been assessed by care professionals, which can be clearly exposed by examining the ways in which this has changed and developed since medieval times. In essence, by looking historically at the development of health and social care we are looking at a case study of the interplay between lay, professional and folk influences within the context of contemporary society or politics. We can also see how the process of care (ASPIRE) has been legitimised or valued as a professional activity within this historical perspective.

The way that vulnerable and marginalised individuals are provided for has a long history and has a significant impact on the way that current provision is organised. From medieval times, vulnerable individuals have been provided for within communities, largely through religious and charitable organisations (Llewellyn *et al.*, 2008). However, when the monasteries were disbanded in the sixteenth century, there was little provision of care and support. The 1601 Poor Law was implemented to provide relief for vulnerable and impoverished people, placing the duty to care within local communities through institutionalised care within parish boundaries (Crawford and Walker, 2008). However, the process of industrialisation and the disparate implementation of policies between parishes led to concerns about the fact that people could too readily receive relief from poverty, which was reducing the work ethic among some poor people. As a result, the 1834 Poor Law Amendment Act was passed, which introduced a system of workhouse provision, based on the less eligibility principle and the deserving/undeserving distinction (Fraser, 1984). This meant that people would enter the workhouse as a last resort and that their condition would be worse than the lowest paid worker providing for their own needs outside the workhouse system. There was no distinction between adults and children in terms of entry into the workhouse, although a system of classification operated within the workhouses, whereby men, women and children were segregated.

Activity

Read *Oliver Twist* by Charles Dickens for a fictional account of conditions in the workhouses. You may also like to watch various film adaptations of this book, although bear in mind that some of these portray a rather romanticised view of the conditions.

What this system of workhouses failed to acknowledge was that the processes of industrialisation and urbanisation had created structural inequalities, leading to inability to work and be independent because of sickness and disability among a significant percentage of lower paid workers. Thus the workhouses were populated with large numbers of sick and diseased people, who became housed separately in workhouse infirmaries. At the same time, large numbers of people with mental health problems also populated the workhouses, and medical provisions for these people tended to be the largest item of workhouse expenditure (Pelling *et al.*, 1993). Thus, in the 1860s, large-scale asylums were built to house people who were seen as mentally ill and mentally defective.

This development was significant as it had the effect of categorising people according to differing needs, and providing for these needs within segregated institutions. This has contemporary relevance as, although a process of deinstitutionalisation has occurred (see Chapters 2 and 8), delivery of health and social care continues to be provided on this basis of the classification of need and categorisation of individuals.

The voluntary hospitals

Alongside the developments in workhouse infirmaries and the asylum system, was the development of voluntary hospitals. These were hospitals that were funded by voluntary contributions, usually through annual donations by subscribers. The source of funding was important, as it reflects a philanthropic approach to health care, which determined who would be admitted to and treated within the voluntary hospitals. Admission was restricted to people who were seen as 'deserving', reflecting the deserving/undeserving ideology of the Poor Law. People could be admitted if they had a letter of support from a subscriber, which created a dependence of the poor on the goodwill of the rich. Throughout the nineteenth century, the voluntary hospitals became increasingly selective in who they would admit, and the focus was very much on people with acute problems to the exclusion of those with chronic health problems (Ham, 2009).

These developments in hospital-based health care were significant in the perpetuation of medical control over health and illness. As treatments and diagnoses developed, medicine became increasingly focused on objective and empirical measures, and the patient became increasingly passive in the medical encounter (Hardey, 1998). Thus, assessment of health needs was carried out by medical practitioners, who gained increased respectability within their communities. Although doctors principally operated as private practitioners on a fee-for-service basis, the occupation was becoming more worthy and practitioners redefined themselves as General Practitioners, giving a further air of authority and respectability. Medical practice also became more exclusionary, with the establishment of the General Medical Council under the 1858 Act which allowed for restricted access into the profession and established a required programme of training for doctors (Allsop, 1984).

Welfare reforms of the twentieth century

At the start of the twentieth century there was increasing acknowledge-ment that people may require support for poverty and pauperism that is beyond their control. This had an impact on the funding of health care, as a period of legislative activity, known as the liberal welfare reforms, at the turn of the twentieth century introduced the insurance principle for health care. In 1911 Lloyd George, the Chancellor of the Exchequer, observed that although some people had made some provision to cover any period of ill health, this was often inadequate and that there was a high cost to the treasury of providing for people who had either no cover or inadequate cover. Thus, the National Insurance Act (1911) introduced health insurance for some working men, although it operated within strict constraints (Laybourn, 1995).

It was not until there was an ideological change, which occurred during World War Two with a growing acknowledgement that welfare services should be provided to promote a more equal and socially just society, that health care provision became more universal. This was encapsulated in the Beveridge Report (1942) where William Beveridge set out his vision for welfare state provision, in which he identified five areas of serious need within Britain as want, disease, ignorance, squalor and idleness. Following this, the creation of a welfare state was proposed. This was to set a standard below which no citizen should be allowed to fall and the National Health Service Act of 1946 led to the creation of the NHS in July 1948 primarily to address the area of disease. This resulted from an increasing recognition of the need for industrialised societies to provide both an infrastructure that enabled a healthy workforce and a safety net for those who were unable to earn a living independently due to ill health, learning disability or caring commitments. Put bluntly, a healthy workforce or armed force (in addition to elements such as transport systems, energy, etc.) is a functional requirement of an economic system, the recognition of which, it has been argued, eventually led to the development of the welfare state as we see it now (Crinson, 2008).

The National Health Service

After World War Two, the NHS was established to provide free health care to all citizens, irrespective of their ability to pay.

> The first health system in any Western society to offer free medical care to the entire population . . . it was a unique example of the collectivist principle of health care in a market society.
>
> (Klein, 2005:1)

The hospitals were nationalised and health care was predominantly funded through general taxation (Midwinter, 1994). In addition to being based on universalist and collectivist principles, where people's health care needs would be addressed from cradle to grave, the new NHS provided doctors with professional accountability. This firmly located authority for clinical decision-making within their hands, further reinforcing the dominance of the biomedical model within health care provision and the assessment of health needs.

The introduction of the NHS did not happen unfought and there was rigorous opposition from the medical professions who feared loss of independence, professional status and financial loss. Therefore, many concessions were made allowing medical practitioners to retain a privileged position, with GPs remaining as independent contractors and Hospital Consultants retaining their private practice while working in the NHS. These anomalies remain contentious and difficult to this day.

Successive governments have struggled to convince the public that the NHS is safe in their hands. The administrative function has been contentious; different attempts have been made to manage the huge bureaucratic organisation and funding has continued to be a major political pressure. However, a significant proportion of Gross Domestic Product (GDP) (the total value of all goods and products made within a year as a measure of a country's economic performance) has been committed to running the NHS. In 2007, £118 billion (8.4 per cent of GDP) was spent on health care (Office for National Statistics, 2009), but there continues to be criticism of under-funding, over-funding and waste in the running of the NHS. In 1979, the *Merrison Commission Report* (followed by the *Black Report*, 1980) reported widening social and geographical health inequalities, despite the existence of the NHS, further questioning the claims of effectiveness and efficiency. The then Conservative Government responded to this by criticising, through the *Griffiths Inquiry Report* (DHSS, 1983), the form of consensus management favoured by doctors working in the NHS and, in the mid-1980s, the principle of general management was introduced into the NHS. This was to challenge the ethos of the NHS as professionally led, with a lack of sanctions on hospitals with above average costs, which had failed to provide the incentives necessary for staff to achieve any form of efficiency.

Developments in social care

Provision of social care is concerned with addressing social issues, such as welfare, social work with children and older people, addressing the effects of poverty, and personal needs such as personal hygiene needs, shopping and cleaning. However, these needs are much more difficult to define and assess, and the history of social care developments is much more nebulous than the history of health care developments.

Within the programme of legislation and welfare reform in this post World War Two era, provision was made to improve the shelter, education and nutrition of the British population. Plans were made to improve the stock of housing as well as the quality of the current housing stock to reduce squalor, and proposals to improve the education of all children aged up to 15 (with recommendations to increase this to 16) were implemented under the 1944 Education Act to tackle Beveridge's giant of 'ignorance' (Glennester, 1995). Nutrition was improved through the systems of rationing and food allocation that lasted until the mid-1950s and full employment was promoted through a system of nationalised industries and demand management of the economy under Keynesian economic policies to reduce idleness (Jones, 1994).

In the post World War Two reorganisation of welfare, responsibility for personal social services to address social needs was incorporated into the Department of Health and Social Security (which became the Department of Health in 1982). The day to day running of social services was the responsibility of Local Authorities and, later, the Social Services Departments (SSDs) that were established in 1970/71 as a result of the Seebohm Reorganisation (Barclay Report, 1980). These SSDs united disparate services for vulnerable groups including children, mothers and babies, people with disabilities (physical and learning) and older people.

Developments in personal social services and social care operated alongside the development in health care services, although the historical development of these services, with the emphasis on institutional care and medical hegemony (dominance of the system of care by a medical approach to treatment), led to inequalities in power between health and social care services and a continuing institutionalised approach. However, post World War Two, there were also developments in welfare support for vulnerable adults, with the introduction of welfare officers whose role was to deliver personal care services through a variety of providers from the voluntary sector and local authority services that had largely developed through the Poor Law (Crawford and Walker, 2008). Children's Welfare Officers were also appointed to staff newly formed Children's Departments within the Local Authority, formalising the different classification and management of children's services.

Health and social care in the twenty-first century

Payne (2006) identifies four distinct periods in provision for social needs. Up until the end of the nineteenth century, social needs were provided for in institutions (see discussion about the Poor Law above). At the start of the twentieth century, there was increased commitment to the development of community-based responses to social needs, with a distinct shift in ideological commitment to community-based responses during the 1960s and 1970s, with a number of government papers and advisory documents stating the argument for community care and provision. This culminated in the legislative processes of the 1980s and 1990s, with emphasis on assessment of individual needs, as identified in the 1990 NHS and Community Care Act, with the two main aims of maximising independence and providing choice of services (see Chapter 2). A key part of this emphasis on choice was the provision of services from different provider agencies, including private and third sector providers as well as statutory services.

The responsibility for personal and social needs is located at government level within the Department of Health, and local authority social service departments administer personal social care, but the reality of provision is that there is a mixed economy of welfare (Webb and Wistow, 1982), reflecting successive governments' policy imperatives to increase service user choice and to improve the efficiency of services. Alongside local authority social service department provision, personal social care is also provided by voluntary organisations, private providers and through informal care arrangements by relatives, friends and neighbours. Evers *et al.* (1994) refer to this as the Welfare Diamond, with the care recipient at the centre of this mixed economy.

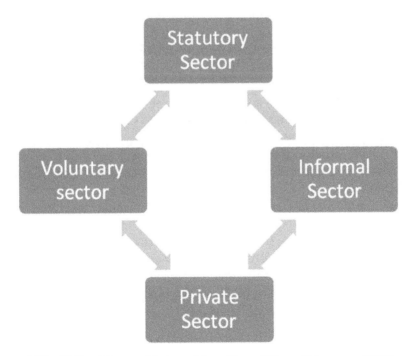

Figure 3 The Welfare Diamond (adapted from Evers, Pijls and Ungerson, 1994)

This model of care theoretically provides care recipients with choices about the provision of services. However, Webb and Wistow (1982) have argued that this mixed economy of welfare actually limits the scope of statutory care provision, as it can be substituted by other forms of provision. The professional health or social care practitioner within the statutory sector of care makes up a very small proportion of the whole health and social care workforce, and care (particularly personal care) is increasingly provided by lower paid and lower qualified personnel within either the statutory or private sectors or by unqualified (and often unpaid) carers within the voluntary and informal sectors.

> More than 1 million people are employed in the care workforce in Britain – over 750,000 in social care and nearly 350,000 in childcare. They are mostly women (88 percent), especially in childcare, and, apart from social workers, they have below average levels of qualifications.
>
> (Simon *et al.*, 2003)

This has implications both in terms of funding for statutory services and in terms of the relative importance placed on social care in relation to health care. Although personal care services are administered by the same government department as health services, it has been argued that social needs have not been seen as being as significant as health needs, and there has been more emphasis on the resourcing of services to address these health needs, reflecting the power and domination of the biomedical model of health care (Horner, 2009).

The development of health and social care policies prior to the 1900s was therefore based on the mass incarceration of the vulnerable in institutions (generically at first, but later in specialist, segregated institutions). The legacy of this is that a system of classification was developed that formed the basis for contemporary policy ideas about separate service user groups. In addition, a welfarist model of health and social care developed, with professional power and service-led provision dominating. However, we have also witnessed unequal professional power relationships developing with a medical hegemony (dominance) of health and social care provision. Although a process of deinstitutionalisation and normalisation has been implemented since 1990, this medical hegemony arguably still exists, leading to potential conflicts between the medical and the social model in provision for many vulnerable groups.

The historical development paths of health and social care services have therefore differed, leading to organisationally separate services, which lack shared geographical boundaries, leading to barriers in collaborative working. This has been further exacerbated through increasing problems of budgetary limitations in a financially constrained service, where demand will always outstrip supply. Funding of health and social care has also been separated, with health care being funded through taxation policies, and therefore being free at the point of need, while social care has been funded on the basis of eligibility criteria, determined by level of need and ability to pay. Lymbery (2005) has referred to a Berlin Wall between health and social care, with the '"Absolute" rights of health care versus "contingent" rights of social care' (Salter, 1998), leading to further potential conflict and difficulties in cooperation between agencies (see Table 3). This has impacted on the assessment, planning and implementation phases of the ASPIRE process. Although the reality for the service user is that health and social care needs are difficult to separate as they impact on one another, the reality in terms of provision is that these important functions have been separated, leading to an inadequate process of assessment and fragmentation in the planning and implementation of care. For example, duplication and repetition of assessments for older people with complex care needs may have been a reflection of the multiple assessments carried out by different professionals. On the other hand, they may have fallen through the gap in services, with professionals believing that a different occupational group was addressing their needs.

Activity

May, aged 84, has a leg ulcer that needs to be treated and dressed twice weekly. She also has limited mobility and requires help with washing and dressing. The district nurse visits twice weekly to dress her leg ulcer, and a social care assistant visits daily to help May to wash and dress.

1. What are the implications of this for the quality of care that May receives?
2. Do you think that this is an efficient use of health and social care resources?

The 1990 NHS and Community Care Act has been significant in changing the direction of health and social care policy, and can be seen partly as a response to a changing health and social care environment. Nettleton (2006) identifies transformations in health care, associated with demographic change and the rise in chronic illness, making the traditional curative model of health care less effective. Developments in health and social care in the twenty-first century have therefore acknowledged these

	Health care institutions	Social care institutions
Institutional/ financial:	Free at point of use.	Responsibility of individuals or means tested.
Rights	Social right.	Residual right.
Level of government:	National.	Local.
Professional orientation:	Medicine and professions ancillary to medicine.	Social work.
Professional status:	Accepted.	Disputed.
Knowledge base:	Bioscience (hard).	Social science/ therapeutics (soft).
Application of technology:	High and esteemed.	Low and not esteemed.
Action:	Direct – bodily.	Vague – psychosocial.
Legitimation and power:	'Real' life and death needs. Necessary.	More disputed 'needs'. Optional.

Table 3 The medical/social boundary in health and social care (adapted from Baldock et al., 2007)

transformations, and contemporary policies and provisions emphasise the need for collaborative person-centred care (DH, 2006a), with a focus on the holistic needs of the care recipient.

HOLISTIC CARE

Although the medical and social models of health and illness both have important elements within them, it is increasingly recognised that a holistic concept, amalgamating elements of the two models, provides the most comprehensive approach to both understanding and delivering health and social care (see Figure 4). Holistic care is defined as the inter-relationship between biological, psychological and social factors (Hockley and Clark, 2002); while for Patterson (1998) holistic care encompasses elements of mind, body and spirit.

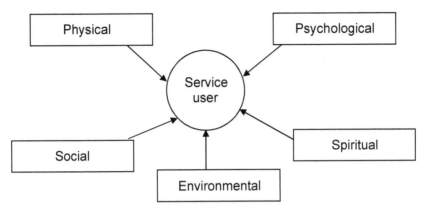

Figure 4 A diagrammatic representation of holistic care

The World Health Organisation (WHO) acknowledged the complexity of health and the inter-relationship of the different elements in its 1984 definition of health.

> The extent to which an individual or group is able, on the one hand, to realize aspirations and satisfy needs and on the other hand, to change or cope with the environment. Health is therefore seen as a resource for everyday life, not the objective of living: it is a positive concept emphasizing social and personal resources as well as physical capabilities.
>
> (WHO, 1984)

It is increasingly acknowledged that health and social care are complex and multidimensional concepts and that there is a need for a holistic approach to care that addresses both health and social needs, with agencies working in partnership to provide packages of care that address individual need. Services have historically developed according to a welfarist model, where welfare professionals have identified needs and then provided services to address these needs (see the discussion above about normative need). The change in the nature of illness and an increase in consumerism and consumer rights has led to a shift in ideology and power, with greater emphasis on user and carer involvement in care and individual assessment of need and care packages tailored to meet those needs. A consumerist approach to health and illness sees care as a commodity, which can be bought and sold, leading to greater control and choice for care recipients (Leece, 2004). Thus there is a shift from service-led provision to needs-led care, with the care recipient at the centre of the decision-making process. There is a much greater emphasis on 'self-help' or 'self-health' based on the ways in which people take responsibility for their own health and motivate themselves to avoid or manage illness. This can include lifestyle choices such as diet, exercise and relaxation, or health care choices such as complementary and alternative therapies. This reflects the greater emphasis on individual resources and how these can be used to promote wellbeing.

The Single Assessment Process and The Recovery Model of mental health are good examples of this shift in emphasis. For both of these models, the starting point of assessment is the service user and their perception and identification of their needs, and care is assessed and planned with the service user central to the decision-making process, emphasising their strengths and coping strategies (Repper and Perkins, 2003; DH, 2002a). The focus therefore shifts from cure to prevention and changing the balance between health and social care services.

This shift in ideology and balance of provision of services has led to a need for more collaborative and partnership working between the different professional groups involved in the delivery of health and social care and with service users and carers (see Chapter 5).

SUMMARY

This chapter has set the scene for ASPIRE within health and social care by starting with the definitions of health and social care. This has enabled you to understand the historical context of the development of health and social care as concerns of the policy-makers, professionals and individuals within society. Definitions of health and health behaviours were explored and the historical development of health and social care examined with reference to the biomedical and social models of health care. The chapter also considered the importance of user and carer perspectives in health and social care delivery, exploring the concept of power within these relationships. It traced the origins of the care process by examining the role of the individuals and their specific roles as 'service user', 'carer' or 'professional practitioner'. The relationship between health and social care was also scrutinised emphasising the problems caused by separating health and social care provision and thus the importance of joint working between health and social care agencies in the provision of person-centred care.

Reflection	
Identify at least three things that you have learned from this chapter.	1. 2. 3.
How do you plan to use this knowledge within care practice?	1. 2. 3.
How will you evaluate the effectiveness of your plan?	1. 2. 3.
What further knowledge and evidence do you need?	1. 2. 3.

FURTHER READING

Brotherton, G. and Parker, S. (2007) *Your Foundation in Health & Social Care: A Guide for Foundation Degree Students*. London: Sage

Written to accompany the Foundation degree in Health and Social Care, and other higher education courses in the same area, this book gives the reader the knowledge and skills necessary for effective learning both in academia and in the workplace. It includes case studies drawn from a range of health and social care settings to illustrate 'real-life' practice. Suggested essay topics, activities and further research features encourage the reader to develop their knowledge and understanding. The study skills tips and guidelines for approaching learning are also useful.

Johnson, J. and De Souza, C. (2009) *Understanding Health and Social Care: An Introductory Reader*. London: Sage

This excellent book covers the key issues in health and social care. The material includes the voices of service users, professional and lay carers, as well as academics and researchers. It is organised into four sections, each with a section introduction pulling together the main themes:

People
- focuses on those who use and provide health and social care services;

Places
- focuses on where care takes place;

Approaches
- considers different ways in which care takes places;

Ideas
- focuses on the ideas and policies that underpin care provision.

It has real practice scenarios and examples to help the reader to make the link between theory and practice.

Nettleton, S. (2006) *The Sociology of Health and Illness*. Cambridge: Polity

This is a well-written, engaging and theoretically-informed discussion of health sociology in modern Britain. It blends relevant classical and contemporary theories into an explanation of key concepts and issues and provides a lively, balanced and up-to-date introduction to medical sociology. It also discusses issues of interest to health economists, health services researchers and health care policy-makers. The sections on definitions of health and the changing nature of health care delivery are of particular relevance.

Chapter 2

The Politics and Key Policy Drivers in Health and Social Care

---

This chapter covers the following key issues:

- the current and evolving context for health and social care services;
- definitions of policy;
- the policy-making process;
- factors that influence policy and policy-making;
- the ways that policy affects the process of ASPIRE in health and social care.

By the end of this chapter you should be able to:

- discuss health and social care policy;
- understand the factors that influence policy and policy-making;
- describe the key contemporary policy themes that drive health and social care policy and provision;
- understand why policy is so important to the care process.

This chapter matches to the following National Occupational Standards and Essential Skills Clusters:

- ESC 1.iii Promotes a professional image.
- NOS 18.1 Review and update your own knowledge of legal, policy and procedural frameworks;
- NOS 21.1 Contribute to policy review and development.

INTRODUCTION

Health and social care services take place within a political and ideological context, which is constantly evolving and which, in the twenty-first century, takes place on a global stage. At the time of writing the New Labour Government that has shaped health and social care policy over the last 13 years has ended and a new Conservative/Liberal Democratic Coalition Government is in power. It is too early to assess the impact of this political change, although it is already clear that health and social care provision will be subject to financial review and the policy changes which result from this will become apparent over the coming months and years. This chapter will therefore explore the current and evolving context for health and social care services by defining policy, introducing the factors that influence policy and policy-making and finally setting out the current key policy drivers that drive health and social care service provision acknowledging that these policy drivers are constantly evolving. The explicit link between health and social care policy and the experience of individual practitioners and care recipients working and receiving care within health and social care services, and when engaged within the care process, will be demonstrated and linked clearly to the ASPIRE process. One clear example of policy that has made an impact is the Government's approach to reducing the burden on public health of smoking (DH, 2004a). This policy has been publicly debated and has impacted in many ways on health and social care provision as well as on society in general as seen on legislation banning smoking in public places.

Activity

1. Think about how the policy on smoking has impacted on the following individuals.
2. Identify the ways in which their health and social care needs are met.

Case study 1

Ivy is 86 and has smoked for 73 years. She lives in a local authority care home and is unable to get outside independently.

Case study 2

Gemma is 21 and has brittle asthma. Before the smoking ban was introduced, she spent time with her Practice Nurse planning how she could self-care and avoid situations that would aggravate her condition. Part of the agreed plan was not to enter smoky atmospheres as this may set off an asthma attack. She did tell her Practice Nurse that she is actually frightened to go into a pub with her friends, as the last time she did she had to leave as she was having difficulty with her chest feeling tight and experiencing shortness of breath.

Case study 3

Jane is a Practice Nurse. She is an ex-smoker and has wanted to set up a 'quit smoking' clinic for a number of years as she feels that there is little formal provision of services for individuals wanting to quit.

These very brief case studies illustrate the impact of health policy at both service and individual level. Ivy and the manager of her care home will now contend with legislation that bans smoking in public places and in property that is owned and managed by care services. This raises questions about how the home will address this issue and ensure that they are able to meet Ivy's assessed needs in a planned way. Perhaps they may assess her and decide the best option is for Ivy to quit smoking, or the assessment of her need may be that it would be too difficult for her to quit. Could they therefore plan to provide a smoking area outside the property or would the law allow smoking inside the resident's bedroom as she lives in a residential home? There are implications of implementing either of these plans, in terms of Ivy's freedom of choice or her socialising within the day areas or the dangers of smoking in a bedroom, isolated from staff and other residents.

The case for Gemma is far less contentious. She is now able to go to her local pub in the knowledge that she will not be exposed to tobacco smoke and so the implementation of part of her planned self-care package is achievable.

In terms of service provision the policy of reducing smoking in the population as a whole is a great relief to Jane. She had tried unsuccessfully through the 1990s to set up a 'quit smoking' clinic but now, due to increased funding for smoking services, she can access funding through her local Primary Care Trust to set up a local clinic. She also has a number of services that she can refer smokers to if they prefer not to attend the GP Surgery for their 'quit smoking' advice. This includes stop smoking clinics, brief intervention services, access to medication to help the addiction (patches and tablets) and there is even a 'smoke free houses' service that will visit families to advise on keeping homes free of smoke.

These case studies demonstrate how policies affect individuals and societies and how they influence decisions about assessment, planning and implementation of care. But what is policy and who decides on which policies are introduced?

DEFINING POLICY

Policy is simply a deliberate plan of action that is intended to achieve specific outcomes. Policy-making is fundamentally a political process and involves organisational processes and decision-making structures in initiating, creating and implementing any policy decision. The policy-making process is thus made up of key policy actors, usually politicians and political parties, pressure groups and policy networks who have to a greater or lesser extent the capacity or power to influence the policy decision-making process. The policy-making process also makes reference to an economic context, in terms of what is affordable and what should be prioritised, which, of course, has huge implications for the ASPIRE process in terms of which services are funded and therefore what provision can be planned and accessed.

Within the British political system of government, politicians, along with their advisors, set out policy proposals that are based on the political values and ideology of their political party and these are set out in election manifestos (Crinson, 2008). These political programmes are democratically put to the electorate and the political party whose programme is supported by the majority of the population who voted forms a government. Once in power the party sets out its legislative programme and then a formal process of consultation occurs where pressure groups can lobby for their views to be incorporated. Pressure groups are groups of interested individuals who form together to promote a particular objective (for example, the banning of fox hunting). A number of different pressure groups, reflecting different interests and objectives, may lobby on a particular issue, and their degree of influence may be related to their relative power (Punnett, 1994). The final detailed proposals are then set out in a 'White Paper' and a final parliamentary debate occurs following which the House of Commons votes and an Act of Parliament (legislation) is then passed.

This balance of public choice, political party politics and interest or pressure groups works out the policy process, supported by the politically neutral bureaucratic organisation, staffed by civil servants, who support the process. It is of course argued that the civil servants themselves wield large political power as separate from the political parties but, mindful

Activity

Think about the policies relating to the reduction of the incidence of smoking in the UK.

1. Using the Department of Health website can you find a policy document that makes reference to reducing the incidence of smoking?
2. What legislation followed this policy?
3. Can you name a pressure group that supports the ban on smoking in public places and one that is opposed to it?

of issues such as fiscal balance, the civil servants are able to contribute to the policy-making process through their provision of 'expertise' and their contributions to policy decisions during both their creation and implementation.

Policy implementation

Policy implementation is a very complex process often marked with a series of negotiations and compromises. In fact policies are highly complex and can involve purely symbolic elements alongside practice elements which politicians have no intention of actually implementing (Crinson, 2008).

Top-down approaches to policy implementation, which are guided by authority and policy directives to ensure a successful 'rolling out' of policy, often fail if there is a failure by policy-makers to engage the organisations with the political goals of the policies. Bottom-up models, where trust is placed in those implementing the policy in order for them to have freedom to handle uncertainties associated with new policies, carry much greater realism and success by allowing more spontaneity and problem-solving in contrast to the control, minute planning and hierarchy of top-down approaches.

THE POLITICAL CONTEXT OF THE HEALTH AND SOCIAL CARE SERVICES

Community care policy

Throughout the latter half of the twentieth century there were growing concerns about the nature of institutionalised care for vulnerable people, and the way in which the needs of vulnerable people were assessed, planned and implemented within this context. A series of proposals were therefore made in relation to community care policy. These various documents culminated in the legislation of the National Health Service and Community Care Act (DH, 1990), which came into force in 1993 (Means, Richards and Smith, 2008).

Activity

Think about the way care was delivered in the 1970s and 1980s before the Community Care Act was introduced.

1. How were the needs of vulnerable individuals with severe and enduring mental health needs assessed and care planned and implemented in large institutions for 'inpatients'?
2. How does that contrast with care today when individuals are supported in the community?

The 1990 NHS and Community Care Act (NHSCCA) built on the proposals outlined in the 1989 White Paper, which identified six key objectives in service delivery and design.

- To promote the development of domiciliary, day and respite services to enable people to live in their own homes wherever feasible and sensible (*essentially improving how care could be planned and implemented*).
- To ensure that service providers make practical support for carers a high priority (*essentially supported the implementation of informal care arrangements*).
- To make proper assessment of need and good care management the cornerstone of high quality care (*reviewing and improving assessment methods*).
- To promote the development of a flourishing independent sector alongside good quality public services (*offering alternative models to and places of care implementation*).
- To clarify the responsibilities of agencies and so make it easier to hold them to account for their performances (*enabling better planning and evaluation of care*).
- To secure better value for taxpayers' money by introducing a new funding structure for social care.

(Department of Health, 1989a, para 1.11 – authors'
additions in italics to demonstrate the relationship
between the objectives of the Act and the ASPIRE process.)

The NHS and Community Care Act (1990) (NHSCCA) did not consolidate previous legislation but provided an umbrella framework for the organisation and delivery of services, with an emphasis on community-based care, a needs-led service rather than service-led provision, an emphasis on working in partnership with independent sector providers and a shift in funding from the NHS to local government (Ham, 2009). Local authorities were given commissioning powers, including joint commissioning with NHS providers, with the proviso that 85 per cent of funding should be used to purchase independent care services. The Act introduced the concept of care management, which includes the whole process of assessment for services, as well as provision and review and evaluation of services. In addition, under section 47 of the Act, service users were given the right to assessment of need for community care services:

> where it appears to a local authority that any person for whom they may provide or arrange for the provision of community care services may be in need of such services, the authority
>
> a. shall carry out an assessment of his needs for those services; and
> b. having regard to the results of that assessment, shall then decide whether his needs call for the provision by them of any such services.
>
> (DH, 1990: section 47[1])

Section	Summary
46	Community care plans.
46(3)	Definition of community care services.
47	Assessment of need for community care services.
47(5)	Services pending assessment.
48	Inspection of premises where community care services are provided.
50	Complaints procedure.

Table 4 Summary of the key points of the NHS and CC Act (1990)

Caring for People, the White Paper (DH, 1989a) that preceded the Community Care Act (DH, 1990), represented far-reaching policy that proposed a series of radical changes to the structure of health and social care provision. This came to be known as internal market reform and essentially aimed to separate the function of purchasing health and social care from the provider function. Hospitals and community services were therefore encouraged to opt out of Health Authority Control and become self-governing Trusts. They then competed with other providers to win contracts from the purchasers of health care, these being the Health Authorities and Fund-holding GP Practices. The belief behind this was that introducing a level of competition would improve efficiency and responsiveness within the health care 'market' (Ham, 2009).

However, the outcome of these reforms left the Labour Government, which came to power in 1997, with a legacy of poor hospital and community health care estates, waiting lists of over 12 months and in some cases 18 months for essential operations such as coronary artery bypass grafts and a deskilled and under-resourced workforce due to underinvestment in the training and professional development of staff (Crinson, 2008).

THE POLICY DIRECTION OF NEW LABOUR (1997–2010)

Shortly after coming to power in June 1997 Frank Dobson, as Secretary of State for Health, issued the policy document *The New NHS – Modern and Dependable* (DH, 1997a), which set out New Labour's initial vision for the NHS. Labour wished 'to rebuild public confidence in the NHS' and set out three main themes, which were:

1. better communication within the service, through initiatives such as developing the NHS Information Technology framework and the nurse-led helpline NHS Direct;
2. an accent upon quality with new national supervisory bodies such as the National Institute for Clinical Excellence and the Commission for Health Improvement (this was later renamed the Health Care Commission and is currently the Care Quality Commission which unites health and social care regulation);
3. a revision of the NHS organisational structure including abolishing the Conservative party-led fund holding, replacing it with the ideals of partnership and 'joined-up thinking' with national guidance stressing the importance of the interdependence of health and social care.

What followed was a decade of unprecedented change at all levels of health and social care services (organisational, clinical and financial). Throughout this period, a succession of reviews led to reforms, modernisation and reorganisation. GP fund holding was replaced with practice-based commissioning, districts became primary health care groups and later Primary Care Trusts, with mergers in 2006 reducing their number to half (152). Ten Regional Health Authorities were divided to create 28 Strategic Health Authorities, which were then merged back into ten Authorities and Foundation Hospital Trusts were created (Crinson, 2008).

Activity

Think about the three main priorities presented in *A New NHS – Modern and Dependable*. How might the ASPIRE process be affected by:

- better communication using the Information Technology Framework?
- the introduction of the nurse-led helpline NHS Direct?
- the introduction of NICE which improved guidance on the use of medicines?
- increased focus on the importance of the interdependence of health and social care?

Just as importantly, however, under New Labour the NHS started to be described or presented as a concept – a concept that is tax-funded, largely free at the point of use, but provided by a variety of organisations. No longer was it a service where provision was only in the public sector facilities that it owned. The service moved from a system in which providers took no risk and service users just waited until they were treated, to one where the search for efficiency spurred a new series of incentives (Rivett, 2009). These changes have been important in relation to the provision of care, as the emphasis has shifted from professionally-led services to a model that places service users at the centre of service provision and allows them to be proactive in the decision-making process in relation to care delivery.

Modernising Social Services

Alongside these developments in health care, a programme of modernisation of social services has taken place. The Audit Commission

Report (1997) argued that there was a need for more proactive preventative services in social care provision to reduce the vicious circle of crisis intervention. This was built on by the White Paper *Modernising Social Services* (DH, 1998a), which set out a vision of a service 'for all of us' (para 1.1) not just for a 'small number of casualties' (para 1.3). This White Paper sets out the key priorities for social work and social care and has formed the basis for development of social care services since 1997. The key priorities can be summarised as follows:

- protection – improvements in safeguards to protect vulnerable children and adults (see Chapter 3);
- co-ordination – improving coordination between different elements of the system;
- flexibility – improving the ability of the service to meet the needs of service users rather than the service providers;
- clarity of role – a focus on expectations and standards;
- consistency – removing geographical inconsistencies in the provision of services across the country;
- efficiency – focusing on minimising cost differentials between different service providers.

(Hatton, 2008)

Activity

Think about some of the main priorities presented in *Modernising Social Services*. How might the ASPIRE process be affected by an increased focus on:

- improved co-ordination between different elements of the system?
- flexibility – improving the ability of the service to meet the needs of service users rather than service providers?
- removing geographical inconsistencies in the provision of services across the country?

At the heart of these priorities and the proposals set out in the White Paper is the imperative to maximise independence, the need to effectively safeguard vulnerable people, to increase public trust and confidence in social workers and social care services, and the need for partnership working within the mixed economy of welfare (see Chapter 1).

Health and social care policies relating to children

Alongside this, there have been radical reforms in children's policies in health and social care, which are located within a wider social context of ideas about children and children's rights and the need for protection and safeguarding of vulnerable children.

In the nineteenth century, there started to be increased state concern about the welfare of children. State concern centred on four broad categories of children:

1. children of the street (beggars, prostitutes, etc.);
2. young offenders;
3. children at work;
4. children looked after by the Poor Law authorities (for example, orphans, children with disabilities, abandoned children, etc.).

(Hobsbawm, 1997)

Since as early as the 1870s, the state has been involved in direct intervention with these categories of vulnerable children and young people, and resources continue to be targeted at these categories of children in the twenty-first century. However, legislation and policy to address concerns was piecemeal and fragmented throughout much of the nineteenth and twentieth centuries. This was addressed under the 1989 Children Act (DH, 1989c), which brought the disparate childcare laws under one single piece of statute, which has been described as 'the most far-reaching reform of the law in living memory' (Lord Mackay, 1989). A series of key principles underpin the Act:

- there should be a new balance of responsibilities for children between parents/carers and the state;
- the former concept of parental rights was replaced by responsibilities and duties;
- children are best brought up in their own families where possible;
- the state should offer support to enable families to bring up their own children, who would be defined as being in need, including children with disabilities;
- if it is not possible to maintain a child at home, then children should be looked after by the state on a temporary basis, on the basis of partnership between the state and parents, with the presumption of family reunification, and ideally on the basis of no court orders being made;
- Local Authorities have a duty to promote and support contact between the child and their family;

- the state should intervene as little as possible;
- due consideration should be given to the child's wishes and feelings and to their religious, cultural, racial and linguistic backgrounds when making decisions and planning interventions.

This mirrors some of the key policy imperatives in adult social care, with the emphasis on rights and service user choice, as well as maximising independence within a community setting. Also, under section 44(7) of the Act, children of sufficient age and understanding were enabled to refuse to undergo medical assessments, acknowledging the rights of children to be involved in the decision-making process about their care (see the discussion of Gillick Competence in Chapter 3).

New Labour politics of the welfare state

New Labour politics represented a radical change from the traditional left-wing politics of the old Left to new 'Third way' politics. This can be described as an attempt to reconcile commitment to social justice with a belief in the operation of a market system to improve efficiency. This is a new approach to politics, which is neither right wing nor left in the traditional sense. Thus, while New Labour remained opposed to the strategies of the Thatcherite era of individualism and the withdrawal of government from the provision of state services, they tried to recast the notions of the need for equality and equity and redistribution of wealth as bedfellows of private market mechanisms. Thus private delivery of services, which increased choice and efficiency, was championed with the belief that it would:

- create consumer involvement and choice;
- stimulate provider rivalry and competition;
- set standards of excellence.

(Bradshaw and Bradshaw, 2004)

This shift in the direction of policy under New Labour has important implications for the delivery of care. The emphasis on consumer involvement and choice is central to contemporary approaches to the assessment, planning, implementation and evaluation of services (see Chapter 3), while the issues of competition and standards of excellence provide a context for choice and value (see Chapters 5 and 6), as well as raising issues about regulation and quality monitoring (see Chapter 7).

Activity

Think about assessing the needs of a client.
How would an emphasis on consumer involvement and choice impact on how the assessment is carried out?

What are the driving forces behind Labour's policy direction?

There are a number of factors that have driven New Labour's policy direction, which demonstrate the complexity of the context of policy decisions. These influencing factors can be summarised as follows:

- demographics;
- the rise in the incidence of Long-Term Conditions;
- technological and pharmaceutical advances;
- globalisation;
- consumerism or the consumer culture;
- a focus on quality (including a focus on 'evidence-based practice');
- funding issues;
- the risk society.

Demographics

A number of demographic changes have taken place in the late twentieth century and early twenty-first century, which have had an impact on the demand and supply of health and social care provision. We live in an ageing society and, on average, older people make greater use of health and social care services than other groups within society (Kings Fund, 2002). While life expectancy has risen significantly in the last 50 years, the birth rate has fallen. The percentage of the population aged under 16 has been declining since 1995 and, for the first time ever, has dropped below the percentage of the population of state pensionable age (Office for National Statistics (ONS), 2008a). Average growth in the population aged over state pensionable age between 1981 to 2007 was less than 1 per cent per year but, between 2006 and 2007, the growth rate was nearly 2 per cent. The fastest growing age group in the population are those aged 80 years and over, who currently constitute 4.5 per cent (2 749 507) of the total population. This age group has increased by over 1.1 million between 1981 and 2007 (1 572 160 to 2 749 507), from 2.8 per cent to 4.5 per cent. This is mainly a result of improvements in mortality at older ages over the second half of the twentieth century (ONS, 2008a). This has significant implications for state funded health and social care services as the current working population pays taxes to support those who have retired. This trend is likely to remain, with the population over state pensionable age continuing to increase, partly due to the number of women born in the immediate post World War Two baby boom who reached state pensionable age in 2007. These women were born in 1947 and the men born in the same year will reach state pensionable age in 2012 (ONS, 2008a). There will therefore be a crisis of funding that will have huge implications for health and social care services and policy changes regarding later retirement ages and the funding of residential and nursing care homes are currently a hotly debated political issue.

Activity

1. What will be the impact of a rising older population on the provision of health and social care services?
2. What policy decisions may the government need to make in order to ensure that health and social care services reach those who need them?

Think particularly about the stages of the ASPIRE process.

There have been other demographic factors that have led to increases in demand for health and social care services. Unemployment is a significant feature of contemporary Western societies (and, more significantly, long-term unemployment), with a causal relationship with both physical and mental health care problems (Bury, 2005). Social exclusion is also a significant feature of contemporary capitalist societies, related to global changes in production, economic changes and the resultant changes in welfare systems. Since the 1970s, there has been a greater emphasis on targeting statutory welfare resources at those most in need, leading to the establishment of eligibility criteria as a means of selectively allocating scarce resources (Parry-Jones and Soulsby, 2001).

Geographical mobility has led to breakdown in communities and kinship networks, impacting on the sense of community and the availability of informal carers within a community care framework. Other spatial processes of segregation and separation such as the increase in travelling communities, the growth in the numbers of refugees and asylum seekers and the growth in homeless and transient populations have all led to social exclusion based on access to the labour market, citizenship rights and social and economic inclusion (Llewellyn *et al.*, 2008).

> We clearly have problems of social exclusion; the proportion of children in workless households is the highest in Europe, more than half the children in inner London are still living below the poverty line, more than 1.2 million young people are not in work or full-time education despite a growing economy, and 2.7 million people of working age are claiming incapacity benefits – three times more than the number who claim jobseeker's allowance.
>
> (Oliver Heald, Conservative Shadow Secretary of State for Constitutional Affairs, 2007, available at **www.egovmonitor.com**)

These factors have led to a change in the constitution of society, affecting the ratio of working populations to non-working populations, which impacts on the funding of health and social care. In addition, community care is partly premised on the notion of people living within established communities, where informal care is provided reciprocally to those who are in need. This breakdown in the nature of community (either as a locality or as a collection of mutually supportive individuals) raises questions about the ideology that underpins community care and makes assumptions about the availability of informal care provision (Llewellyn *et al.*, 2008). This therefore raises questions about the implementation of care within the mixed economy of welfare, which relies on informal care provision. In 2001, 1.2 million men and 1.6 million women aged 50 and over in England and Wales were providing unpaid care to family members, neighbours or relatives. This represents 16 per cent and 17 per cent of older men and women respectively (ONS, 2005). This has implications for the assessment of needs as, under the 2004 Carers (Equal Opportunities) Act (DH, 2004b), carers have to be *informed* of their right to an assessment of their needs, which will then feed into the planning and implementation phases of the care process.

Technological and pharmaceutical advances

In addition to the demographic shift that has led to older people constituting a greater proportion of the population, one of the major policy pressures is the expenditure push associated with innovations in medical technology, the key element of which is the cost of pharmaceuticals (Crinson, 2008). The seemingly exponential rise of the cost of medical technologies somewhat exposes the very naïve assumption made on the establishment of the NHS that there was a fixed amount of illness in society and that sufficient investment of resources would lead to a healthier, i.e. a less 'ill', population and a corresponding reduction in costs. The ageing population receives a year on year increase in the number of prescriptions (DH, 2002c) and make increasing use of novel medical technological improvements that are often more expensive than the procedures they replace (Bradshaw and Bradshaw, 2004). Although the government has attempted to control the use of medicines and technological advances through the publication of guidelines by the National Institute of Health and Clinical Excellence (NICE), these costs continue to rise (see Chapter 7).

The rise in the incidence of Long-Term Conditions (LTCs)

Such demographic changes and medical and technological advances have led to a rise in the incidence of Long-Term Conditions. This refers to the number of individuals living with chronic illnesses such as diabetes, heart disease and chronic obstructive pulmonary disease that can limit lifestyle. There are 15.4 million people living with a long-term condition in England and numbers are expected to rise due to the combination of an aging population and unhealthy lifestyle choices among the population generally (DH, 2009a).

Although the population of Great Britain has been living longer over the past 23 years, the extra years have not necessarily been spent in good health or free from illness or disability. Life expectancy, healthy life expectancy (the expected years of life in good or fairly good health) and disability-free life expectancy (the expected years of life without a limiting illness or disability) all increased between 1981 and 2004 for both men and women, with life expectancy increasing at a faster rate than health expectancy (ONS, 2008b). The difference between life expectancy and health expectancy can be regarded as an estimate of the number of years a person can expect to live in poor health or with a limiting illness or disability. In 1981 the expected time men lived in poor health was 6.5 years. By 2004 this had risen to 8.6 years. Women can expect to live longer in poor health than men. In 1981 the expected time women lived in poor health was 10.1 years, rising to 10.7 years in 2004. The time men can expect to live with a limiting illness or disability has also increased between 1981 and 2004: 12.8 years in 1981 rising to 14.3 years in 2004 (ONS, 2008b).

Therefore, the use of health and social care services varies by age, with individuals in older age groups being more likely to seek medical attention and requiring long-term support for social care needs (Kings Fund, 2002). Ill health and dependence also rises with age. Social care services are therefore affected, with the volume of home help hours purchased or provided by councils in England increasing significantly over the past two decades. In 2004, an estimated 3.4 million contact hours were provided to around 355 600 households. In contrast, 2.2 million hours were provided in 1994. However, while the overall number of hours supplied has increased, the number of households receiving council-funded home care services has fallen consistently since 1994. This suggests that councils are providing more intensive services for a smaller number of households (ONS, 2005).

The impact of LTCs on the NHS and Social Services is highlighted by the DH in their publication *Ten Things You Need To Know About Long-Term Conditions* (see Table 5).

Activity

1. How might the increasing complexity of needs among the ageing population impact on the assessment and planning process?
2. Who needs to be involved?

Globalisation

Another major contextual change is that of increasing globalisation. While globalisation is a complex and multifaceted set of issues it has been summarised by Brotherton and Parker (2007) as a greater connectedness between nation states in a variety of ways.

1. Economic – the rapid movement of jobs and financial resources.
2. Social – increased movement of people through both migration and tourism.
3. Technological – the use of communication technology, such as computers, the internet and mobile phones.

(Brotherton and Parker, 2007: 223)

The impact of globalisation on health and social care services includes issues such as service provision in an increasingly multicultural society, issues about recruitment and training of staff from diverse communities in the UK and the impact of increasing technologies, for example the use of telecare and telehealth (see Chapter 8). It is also argued that globalisation has had a major effect on communities with people no longer living in the same geographical area all of their lives and therefore less able to provide support to ageing relatives and informal care to children (Llewellyn *et al.*, 2008). This has the potential to compound the impact of demographic changes and the availability of informal carers, and could have a further impact on demands made on the welfare state.

1. 15.4 million people in England, or almost one in three of the population, have a long-term condition.

2. Three out of every five people aged over 60 in England have a long-term condition.

3. Due to the aging population, the number of people in England with a long-term condition is set to rise by 23 per cent over the next 25 years.

4. Five per cent of service users with one or more long-term conditions account for 49 per cent of all inpatient hospital bed days.

5. Service users with long-term conditions are intensive users of health care services. Those with long-term conditions account for 31 per cent of the population, but use 52 per cent of all GP appointments and 65 per cent of all outpatient appointments.

6. It is estimated that the treatment and care of those with long-term conditions accounts for 69 per cent of the primary and acute care budget in England.

7. 6.4 million people have clinically identified hypertension. It is estimated that the same number again have unidentified hypertension, meaning that around one in five of the population has the condition.

8. Common mental health problems affect about one in seven of the adult population, with severe mental health problems affecting one in a hundred.

9. The UK economy stands to lose £16 billion over the next 10 years through premature deaths due to heart disease, stroke and diabetes.

10. It is estimated that 85 per cent of deaths in the UK are from chronic diseases. Within this, 36 per cent of all deaths are from cardiovascular disease and 7 percent from chronic respiratory disease.

**www.dh.gov.uk/en/Healthcare/Longtermconditions/
tenthingsyouneedtoknow/index.htm** (last accessed 18.8.09)

Table 5 Ten Things You Need To Know About Long-Term Conditions

Consumerism or the consumer culture

It can be argued that we live in a consumer society where individual demand is key. Consumer power lies within the demand-led market. Within the public services, consumerism is used to argue for the rights of service users to greater participation in the decisions that affect their lives (Crinson, 2008) (see Chapter 5).

Activity

How might increasing consumerism affect how individual health and social care practitioners assess, plan, implement and evaluate an individual's care needs?

Consumerism and practices of consumption are important elements of advanced capitalist society, with the commodification of goods and services. This commodification process can be linked to developments in the global economy and the way in which these reflect the priorities of the more powerful nations.

There has been a change in public attitudes and expectations as health and social care services have come to be seen as a right of individuals, reflecting the consumerist paradigm. Allsop (1984) argues that these expectations are related to the increased availability of information about health and social care services, as well as providers' own successes in promoting their services. It has been argued that the universalist approach of health care services has led to a dependency on medical professionals, with the assumption that we can be consumers of services for treatment, prevention and rehabilitation.

Activity

How would the expectations of an individual being assessed for health and social care needs vary, depending on whether they feel dependency or gratitude for the services of the care professions, or whether the consumer expects access to service provision?

The role of informal care

Informal care provided by families and friends has always been an important part of health and social care delivery (see Chapter 1). However, the third way politics of the New Labour governments has served to further strengthen the role of informal care within the mixed economy of welfare (Evers *et al.*, 1994). Alongside this, there has been a policy shift from providing payments to carers to providing payments to care users (see the section on personalisation and self-directed support in Chapter 3). Within this care system, individuals are empowered to pay for their own packages of care, fundamentally shifting the relationship between the family, the market and the state. This, in turn, challenges the organisation of health and social care where provision is medicalised, professionalised and bureaucratised. There is a further challenge to the gift relationship (Cheal, 1988), where care is provided within the context of a personal relationship, as the care becomes commodified within the market economy of provision. However, despite this change in the nature of care provision, caring remains gendered, with women continuing to provide much of the care within both the formal and informal sectors of the health and social care system (Ungerson, 1997). This raises further issues about the assessment of carers' needs and their ability to provide care within the mixed economy of welfare.

Quality

In addition to the need for government to be accountable for the efficiency and effectiveness of health and social care services and following a number of health care disasters in the 1980s and 1990s (The Bristol Inquiry, 2001; the Allitt Report (DH, 1993); Harold Shipman (HMSO and DH, 1999) and child deaths in the 1990s and 2000s (Victoria Climbié in February 2000 and Baby Peter in August 2007)) have meant that the Government is under pressure to ensure that such incidents which damage public confidence are addressed. As a result there is a raft of quality measures that impact on health and social care and the policy emphasis on evidence-based practice is one example of this. This will be explored in detail in Chapter 7.

Key policy themes

These key factors which impact on the context of care have resulted in key policy themes within health and social care that can be discussed in five areas: Patients, Prevention, Performance, Professional and Partnership, all underpinned by a shift towards moving care more into the community.

Patients (service users)

Although the ideology of prioritising user choice and decision-making can be found within health and social care White Papers that stretch back over two decades to the early years of the Conservative administration under Prime Minister Margaret Thatcher (Crinson, 2008), 'patient power' started to rise to the forefront following the introduction of *Modernising Social Services* (DH, 1998a) and *The NHS Plan* (DH, 2000a) by New Labour. Practical elements such as the establishment of Patient Advisory and Liaison Services (PALS) were introduced to provide assistance to service users, with the aim of resolving complaints where possible but helping service users when a formal complaint seemed appropriate. In September 2001 the Commission for Patient and Public Involvement in Health was introduced, to be replaced in March 2008 by Local Involvement Networks (LINks), which are coterminous with Local Authorities. One hundred and fifty local involvement networks now work with NHS bodies and Local Authorities to involve and consult local communities about changes to services. The membership of these networks includes youth councils, individuals, foundation trust governors, tenants' groups and a wide range of other interests. LINks have the legal right to be consulted about services and, in many instances, to enter premises and inspect services.

Activity

How does external scrutiny through networks such as LINks work to improve the ASPIRE process?

Greater service user choice, which has played an increasing part in New Labour's policy machine, can be seen to be driving the consumerist model that, in turn, drives the reform of the public services and, it is believed, therefore drives quality and equity. This is based on the belief that choice boosts equity as championed by the then Prime Minister Tony Blair in 2003. He described three reasons that choice boosts equity.

1. Universal choice gives poorer people the same choices previously available only to the middle classes, acknowledging that this should address inequities as the lower classes would switch from poor providers. This would need to be a proactive intervention in terms of enabling the poor to access help to explain the range of options to them.

2. Choice sustains social solidarity by ensuring that better off individuals continue to be users of public services.
3. Choice puts pressure on low quality providers to improve performance.

Blair went on to state that choice and consumer power is the route to greater social justice not social division (Blair, 2003).

In December 2003 the Government published a strategy paper *Building on the Best: Choice, Responsiveness and Equity in the NHS*. The proposals included:

- service users having a bigger say in how they are treated and how care is provided – this includes a 'health space' within personal records to make their personal preferences and personal details known to the health and social care team; service users are now able to see doctors' letters about them;
- access to a wider range of services in primary health care, with new providers in areas where primary care had traditionally been weak: nurses to treat more ailments and injuries; commuters might register with a GP near their work while receiving out-of-hours services from their local PCT;
- more choice of where, when and how to get medicines, with a wider role for pharmacies and pharmacists, expanding over the counter remedies and making repeat prescriptions easier to obtain;
- easier hospital appointment booking, with people waiting over six months to be offered alternative provision; ultimately the plan is to lead to patient online booking;
- better service user information using new technology and TV (see Chapter 8).

(Building on the Best: Choice, Responsiveness and Equity in the NHS, DH, 2003a)

By offering choice at the point of GP referral, service users would be given the chance to control their own destiny and to choose the provider that best suited their needs. PCTs were expected to offer service users four or five choices and private/independent care should feature among these.

Activity

How does choice at the point of GP referral impact on the ASPIRE process?

The Green Paper, *Independence, Well Being and Choice* (DH, 2005a), set out proposals for increasing the role of service users and carers in the development and management of social care services, and these were built on in the 2006 White Paper *Our Health, Our Care, Our Say*.

> There will be a radical and sustained shift in the way in which services are delivered – ensuring that they are more personalised and that they fit into people's busy lives. We will give people a stronger voice so that they are the major drivers of service improvement.
>
> Our strategy is to put people more in control, to make services more responsive, to focus on those with complex needs and to shift care closer to home.
>
> (*Our Health, Our Care, Our Say*, DH, 2006a)

The NHS Improvement Plan (DH, 2004d) again championed service user choice as the key point in becoming user-led and described four main goals through which choice would be achieved:

- empowering service users so that they have greater control, especially in terms of the time and place of their care;
- the building of a supply market that allows service users greater choice of where to go (15 per cent of which would be in the private sector);
- the establishment of an information technology system that would enable individuals to become more active in their health and social care, through access to their own records, booking systems and information (see Chapter 5);
- the introduction of a funding system whereby money would follow the patient and so providers of care would be paid a fixed amount for each procedure (Payment by Results – PbR).

Payment by Results

Historically lump sums were paid to individual hospitals, but now payments received by trusts increasingly depend upon the number of cases handled, paid for on the basis of a national tariff. Known as Payment by Results, but really payment by activity, money moves with service users. This was the intention of the Conservative NHS reforms in 1990. In October 2002 the Government issued *Reforming NHS Financial flows – Introducing Payment by Results* (DH, 2002f). A phased programme required PCTs to:

- pay NHS Trusts and other providers on a fair basis while managing demand and risk;
- support patient choice by ensuring that diverse providers were funded according to where service users chose to be treated;
- reward efficiency and quality;
- help match capacity to demand;
- reduce transaction costs and negotiating disputes over price between PCTs and acute Trusts;
- enable PCTs to concentrate on quality and quantity rather than price by setting national tariffs that provide fair prices.

Also, in 2002, the Department of Health published criteria for allocation of funding for community care services, with the aim of providing a more consistent approach to determining eligibility for funding by Local Authorities. This is known as *Fair Access to Care Services (FACS)* (DH, 2002h) and identifies four eligibility bands, based on assessment of need as critical, substantial, moderate and low risk to independence.

Critical risk to independence.	Significant health problems have developed/will develop or serious abuse or neglect has occurred/will occur.
Substantial risk to independence.	There is/will be only partial choice and control over the immediate environment or there is/will be an inability to carry out the majority of personal care or domestic routines.
Moderate risk to independence.	Involvement in several aspects of work, education or learning cannot/will not be sustained or several support systems and relationships cannot/will not be sustained.
Low risk to independence.	There is/will be an inability to carry out one or two personal care or domestic routines or one or two family and other social roles and responsibilities cannot/will not be undertaken.

Table 6 Bands of eligibility in *Fair Access to Care Services* (source: DH, 2002h)

A Patient-Led NHS, published in March 2005 (DH, 2005d), allowed independent providers such as BUPA to be included on the list of choices, and suggested regional or national contracts with providers to reduce the transaction costs of multiple contracts. In January 2006 general implementation began, with patient information leaflets and a website to help people. Service users might now choose private sector hospitals that many thought were cleaner, better managed, had shorter waiting times and provided better facilities.

From April 2008 GPs were able to refer service users to NHS hospitals and some independent sector treatment centres anywhere in England for routine elective treatment. NHS Trusts were able to advertise their services, advertising their waiting times, surgical results and infection rates. Testimonials and sponsorship from appropriate companies would also be permitted (Rivett, 2009).

Activity

How would the patient-focused policy changes described above such as improving choice, setting eligibility criteria and commissioning private providers to deliver NHS services impact on the ASPIRE process?

Prevention

When the NHS was established the principal concern was the treatment of infectious diseases such as Typhoid and TB. Currently the diseases of affluence such as obesity, drug, alcohol and smoking-related illness are a major concern. Underlying this is the recognition that, despite having over 60 years of the NHS, the lower socioeconomic classes have disproportionately higher rates of mortality and morbidity (DH, 2004). As recently as February 2009 the Parliamentary Health Committee reported that while health in the UK was improving, over the last ten years health inequalities between the social classes had widened – the gap has increased by 4 per cent among men, and by 11 per cent among women (Rivett, 2009).

The Improvement Plan (DH, 2004d), like the *NHS Plan* (DH, 2000a) before it, set out a multitude of intentions, one of which was greater concentration on prevention rather than cure. *Health Inequalities: progress and next steps* (DH, 2008) outlined the action being taken within the

NHS, with Primary Care Trusts and Health Trusts instructed to focus on reducing health inequalities as a priority. Local initiatives were started to improve access of minority groups like, for example, Roma populations and pregnant women in areas of deprivation. National targets to reduce inequalities in health outcomes by 10 per cent, as measured by infant mortality and life expectancy at birth, are to be the focus of the commissioning process and new strategies abounded.

Such policy direction can be related specifically to the funding of the NHS. For example, when considering the *Wanless Report* (DH, 2002), ill health prevention can be seen as based on the assumptions about how successful government can be in enabling people in the process of 'protecting and promoting their health and becoming more engaged in managing their health' (DH, 2002, p.1). This scenario is described as 'the fully engaged scenario' and Wanless argues that when the level of 'public engagement in relation to health is high, life expectancy goes beyond current forecasts, health status improves dramatically, use of resources is more efficient' (Wanless, 2004:1).

Activity

Consider the ASPIRE process. How might the policy of increasing the individual's responsibility for their health change the way care is planned and implemented?

Public health interventions also have an influence beyond individuals and ill health prevention goes beyond public health initiatives such as immunisation campaigns, encompassing co-ordination across the government departments. It must include engagement from participants such as voluntary organisations, businesses, service users and carers and community groups (Bradshaw and Bradshaw, 2004) with aims such as:

- improving support for young families and children;
- improving social housing;
- reducing unemployment;
- improving access to public sector services such as NHS and education for disadvantaged groups.

In addition, the prevention of ill health means accepting that with rights to health and social care also come responsibilities, with campaigns and educational initiatives to:

- reduce obesity;
- reduce smoking rates;
- address drugs and addiction;
- increase rates for physical activity.

Activity

Search for information regarding the following government initiatives:

- Sure Start;
- The expert patient programme;
- Fit4life campaign.

1. How successful have they been?

2. What factors have influenced their success?

Professional

On entering power in 1997 the Labour Government did not directly introduce or strengthen the regulation of the health professions but did introduce the professional accountability and quality assurance structure known as Clinical Governance (Crinson, 2008). Based on seven pillars the framework encouraged the use of evidence-based practice and the movement away from routinised practice towards more evidence-based interventions, leading to more efficient and effective practice (see Table 7).

The Health Act (2000) gave the government powers to reform professional regulation without the need to pass new primary legislation and the Department of Health published *Supporting Doctors, Protecting Service Users*, which called for a fundamental review of professional self-regulation and set out 17 principles. *The NHS Plan* (DH, 2000a) outlined the intent to establish a UK Council for Health Care Regulators for the formal co-ordination of professional regulatory bodies. What follows includes a number of initiatives aimed at improving the regulation of all Health and Social Care professions.

The Seven Pillars of Clinical Governance

Clinical effectiveness

Risk management effectiveness

Patient experience

Communication effectiveness

Resource effectiveness

Strategic effectiveness

Learning effectiveness.

Supported by the five foundation stones: systems awareness; teamwork; communication; ownership and leadership.

NHS Clinical Governance Support Team. **(www.cgsupport.nhs.uk/About_CG/ FAQs.asp#seven_pillars)**

Table 7 The Seven Pillars of Clinical Governance

These have been followed up by a number of consultations with professional groups to consider the future of regulation and education – for example:

- Modernising Nursing Careers;
- Modernising Medical Careers;
- the new Degree in Social Work established in 2002, with the intention to 'prepare social workers for the complex and demanding role . . . required of them' (DH, 2002g);
- Children's Workforce Development Council (CWDC) and Skills for Care (SFC) aim to improve care provided to children and adults by ensuring that people working in those areas have the best training, qualifications, support and advice;
- *Fit for Purpose* report (GSCC, 2008a);
- *Raising Standards – Social Work Education in England 2007–8* (GSCC 2009);
- National Social Work Taskforce Review of Social Work Education led by Moira Gibb (DCSF and DH, 2009).

Year	Action
2001	The establishment of the General Social Care Council through the Care Standards Act 2000 to regulate the social care workforce.
2002	Replacement of the United Kingdom Central Council as the regulatory body for nurses and midwives by the Nursing and Midwifery Council and replacement of the Council for Professions Supplementary to Medicine by the Health Professions Council.
2002	The Passage of the NHS Reform and Health Professions Act creates the Council for the Regulation of Health Professions (CHRP) with statutory powers of oversight over the regulators. Medical Act (Amendment) Order 2002 approved enabling introduction of revalidation, new fitness to practise procedures, and changes in governance for GMC.
2003	Establishment of CHRP (now known as the Council for Healthcare Regulatory Excellence). It starts by including performance reviews of all regulatory bodies and development of guidance on how to use its statutory powers.
2004	The General Medical Council introduces new fitness to practise rules with a single complaints process to replace separate conduct, performance, and health proceedings. Shipman Inquiry fifth report extensively reviews both old and new GMC fitness to practise procedures and criticises GMC for failing to protect the public and instead acting in the interests of doctors. Department of Health consults on proposals to establish a new regulatory body for complementary therapies, initially focused on acupuncture and herbal medicine. Department of Health consults on proposals to extend statutory regulation to all healthcare support staff (paralleling the regulation of social care workers by the General Social Care Council).
2007	Government publishes White Paper *Trust, Assurance and Safety – the Regulation of Health Professionals in the 21st Century*, setting out plans for future regulation and followed by legislation.

Table 8 Summary of initiatives aimed at improving the regulation of all health and social care professions (adapted from Rivett, 2009)

Activity

Access your professional body's website.

1. What information can you find about professional regulation?
2. Can you find evidence of practitioners who have been reported and disciplined?
3. What was the nature of their offences?

The social care workforce

The Children's Plan: Building Brighter Futures (DH, 2007c) document highlights the importance of working with children and families in a way that recognises the need to develop integrated and personalised services for children. It builds on work carried out by the *Children's Workforce Strategy* and sets out the plans for the further development of the skills and capacity of the workforce who provide support for children and families.

> Together we want to build a system that provides opportunity and delivers services to meet the needs of children and young people, supports parents and carers, and intervenes early where additional support is needed to get a child or young person back on the path to success. These services need to be delivered by skilled and motivated staff, who achieve excellence in their specialism and work to a shared ambition for the success of every child.
>
> (*The Children's Plan: Building Brighter Futures*, DH, 2007c)

Similarly, the document *Putting People First: A Shared Vision and Commitment to the Transformation of Adult Social Care* (DH, 2007b) states that a new skills academy will be developed in conjunction with key partners in health and social care, in order to ensure appropriate entry level training, continuing professional development and workforce registration so that people working in adult social care are equipped with the appropriate skills and training to meet the challenges posed by changing demography and the transformation of social care services, with the emphasis on personalisation and independent living.

Performance

When Labour entered government in 1997 and published *The New NHS: Modern and Dependable* it stated that:

The new NHS will have quality at its heart. Without it there is unfairness. Every patient who is treated in the NHS wants to know that they can rely on receiving high quality care when they need it. Every part of the NHS, and everyone who works in it, should take responsibility for working to improve quality . . .

(DH, 1997a: 3.2)

Of the six broad principles for the modernisation of health care within this policy one explicitly identified the need to improve quality and a caring service by shifting 'the focus on to quality of care so that excellence is guaranteed to all service users'. The key to this was the underpinning financial necessity to 'improve efficiency so that every pound in the NHS is spent to maximise the care for service users' (DH, 1998b).

Labour's second set of proposals for the NHS was issued in the *NHS Plan* in July 2000 and set out four objectives.

1. **A diagnosis of the problems of the NHS** – including being honest about underfunding.
2. **An identification of priorities** – including increasing capacity, improving responsiveness and dealing with major killing diseases.
3. **Mechanisms to achieve change** – i.e. a focus on the organisation of the NHS.
4. **A broad coalition of interested parties** – a realisation that to make this work NHS staff needed to work together with policy-makers to deliver change.

The NHS Plan was to be long-term, if only because of the time it took to train staff and address issues of public concern such as the need for quicker access to a GP, an end to 'trolley waits' in A&E, booking systems for appointments and treatment, shorter waits for inpatient surgery and better food in cleaner wards. The strategy focused on enhancing the numbers and function of nurses, among a number of other initiatives for which there were details and targets aplenty. These included waiting list targets which meant that service users would not have to wait more than three months to see a specialist, or more than a further six to have an operation, with Trusts meeting these by buying extra capacity, for example by paying their consultants a premium rate to handle additional cases in the evenings or at weekends.

Quality was also to be ensured through the introduction of a whole
raft of other initiatives. Both health and social care organisations
have been historically monitored to ensure quality of performance
by central government. One element of this is independent scrutiny
organisations that, while they are commissioned by central government,
are independent of them. This monitoring has historically been separate,
most recently in health by the Healthcare Commission and in social care
by the Commission for Social Care Inspection and Mental Health Act
Commission. However, as part of the Government's policy to improve
working across the health and social care interface, the Care Quality
Commission (CQC) was established by the Health and Social Care Act
2008 (DH, 2008e). This organisation is now responsible for regulating
the quality of health and social care and looking after the interests
of individuals detained under the Mental Health Act (1983) (CQC,
2008).

At the service level, however, there have been a number of initiatives to
address and improve quality and these include:

1. implementation of professionalism and professional standards;
2. regulation and monitoring through external bodies such as the Care
   Commission and National Institute for Health and Clinical Excellence
   and Social Care Institute for Excellence;
3. use of evidence-based practice (EBP);
4. standard setting and benchmarking;
5. audit;
6. critical incident reporting and safety bulletin reporting;
7. service user surveys and feedback.

See Chapter 7 for a more detailed discussion of these factors.

In 2006, the Department of Health, Social Services and Public Safety set
out its aims for ensuring quality in health and personal social services in
the document *The Quality Standards for Health and Social Care* (DH,
2006). This document sets out standards for quality, with the following
five key quality themes:

- corporate leadership and accountability of organisations;
- safe and effective care;
- accessible, flexible and responsive services;
- promoting, protecting and improving health and social wellbeing;
- effective communication and information.

These standards will be used by the new Regulation and Quality Improvement Authority to assess the quality of care provided by health and personal social services, including regulation of the workforce. Regulation of the quality of care will be linked to the national standard setting bodies of the National Institute for Clinical Excellence (NICE) and the Social Care Institute for Excellence (SCIE) (see Chapter 7).

Partnership

The idea of partnership and collaborative working underpins much health and social welfare policy and legislation in the twenty-first century, identifying the complexities of working across the health and social care interface:

> People remain concerned about poor co-ordination between health and social care services, and want more support for independent living. Overall, the current interface between health and social care appears confusing, lacking in co-ordination and can feel fragmented to the individual.
>
> (*Our Health, Our Care, Our Say*, DH, 2006a: 109)

Similarly, the need for partnership working in relation to children is stressed in various policy documents and legislative processes. In 1991 *Working Together* (DH, 1991), published by the Department of Health, offered guidance to support the Children Act and stressed the importance of agencies working collaboratively together. This was further developed in 2006 in the publication *Working Together to Safeguard Children* (DH, 2006b), with greater emphasis on multi-professional working and consultation (see Chapter 5 for further discussion of partnership and collaborative working).

The role of informal carers

There has also been increased attention paid to the need for health and social care agencies and practitioners to work in partnership with informal carers. *The Carers Strategy* for 2018 sets out the following principles:

- carers will be respected as expert care partners and will have access to the integrated and personalised services they need to support them in their caring role;
- carers will be able to have a life of their own alongside their caring role;
- carers will be supported so that they are not forced into financial hardship by their caring role;
- carers will be supported to stay mentally and physically well and treated with dignity;
- children and young people will be protected from inappropriate caring and have the support they need to learn, develop and thrive, to enjoy positive childhoods and to achieve against all the Every Child Matters outcomes.

(DH, 2009b)

Activity

Consider your role in involving carers in the ASPIRE process.

Funding

The funding of health care

Finally, it is appropriate to consider the issue of funding these policy initiatives. New Labour came into power in 1997 promising to address the historical underfunding of the NHS and increase spending year on year in real terms (i.e. above inflation). Working from a position of prudence, however, the then Chancellor of the Exchequer Gordon Brown simply used the previous Government's spending plans until, in 2001, a major review of health care funding by Derek Wanless was published. *The Wanless Review* (DH, 2002) reported that the country needed to devote a significantly larger share of national income to health care, but that money on its own was not enough – it was essential that resources were efficiently and effectively used. The report saw a wider role for NICE, and an extension of the National Service Frameworks to cover a wider range of diseases. The report set out projections of resources required over the next 20 years, outlining three future scenarios:

1. an optimistic one – the money was wisely and productively used and people demanded better services but learned to look after their own health better;

2. a pessimistic one where people were less involved with health issues and the NHS remained unresponsive;
3. and a middle course in which there was solid progress but not all the desirable changes occurred.

The projections showed the UK spending between 10.6 and 12.5 per cent of GDP on health care by 2022-23, compared with 7.7 per cent in 2002 (DH, 2002).

In response to *The Wanless Review* the 2002 budget committed the government to increased spending on the NHS by 7.4 per cent (real terms) between 2002–3 and 2007–8 in order to reach the average spending by EU countries. Investment was however predicated on reform and thus modernisation became the magic word. There were to be changes in skill mix, using nurses for triage and to replace medical staff, treatment centres, national service frameworks that encouraged transformation, change, improvement and innovation, and a new system of payments – payment by results where the money follows the patient. All this was to be based on the need to accept that all clinical decisions had resource consequences, the need to balance clinical decisions with accountability and support for the systematisation of clinical work.

The funding of social care

The funding of social care remains a contentious issue, with eligibility criteria remaining and resources being targeted at those with the most complex needs, leading to some conflict between health and social care provision (see Chapter 1). Under Part I of the Local Government Act (1999), councils have a duty to provide best value services within a mixed economy of welfare, with the aim of ensuring that the needs of local residents are fully met with the highest possible standard of care. Councils are required to monitor and publish a Best Value Performance Plan, which can be seen within the context of wider bureaucratic requirements of budget setting and commissioning of services.

Activity: The impact of policy on the care of Frank

Refer back to the case study about Frank in Chapter One, pages 19-20.

Reflecting on this chapter, list policies that would have impacted on the way that the care that Frank and his wife needed was delivered through the ASPIRE process.

Many policies will have impacted on the care that both Marjorie and Frank received. The following are examples, although this is not an exhaustive list.

- Marjorie had breast cancer – *The Cancer Plan* (DH, 2000b).
- Marjorie was admitted to hospital – *Essence of Care Benchmarks* from *A First Class Service* (DH, 1998b).
- Frank cared for her at home – *Our Health, Our Care, Our Say* (DH, 2006a), *The Gold Standards Framework* (DH, 2009c), *Independence, Choice and Wellbeing* (DH, 2005a).
- Frank was diagnosed with Type II Diabetes – *The National Service Framework for Diabetes* (DH, 2003b).
- He was able to see a dietitian at the local health centre – *Our Health, Our Care, Our Say* (DH, 2006a).
- Frank also has essential hypertension, which is controlled with an angiotensin converting enzyme (ACE) inhibitor – *The NSF for Coronary Heart Disease* (DH, 2000c), The NICE Guidelines.

You may wish to download the executive summary of one of these policy documents from the Department of Health website (**www.dh.gov.uk**) and examine more closely how it relates to the ASPIRE process.

SUMMARY

This chapter has examined the current and evolving context for health and social care services relating this directly to the process of ASPIRE. It did this by firstly defining policy and then examining the factors that influence policy and policy-making. The factors that were examined were: demographics; technological and pharmaceutical advances; the rise in the incidence of Long-Term Conditions; globalisation; consumerism or the consumer culture; the increasing focus on quality (including evidence-based practice); the impact of funding. Key contemporary policy themes that drive health and social care service policy and provision were then examined including: the service users; prevention of health and social care needs; performance; the role of the professions and their regulation; partnership. Through this approach the importance of policy-making and its relationship to implementation of the care process has been demonstrated.

Reflection	
Identify at least three things that you have learned from this chapter.	1. 2. 3.
How do you plan to use this knowledge within care practice?	1. 2. 3.
How will you evaluate the effectiveness of your plan?	1. 2. 3.
What further knowledge and evidence do you need?	1. 2. 3.

FURTHER READING

Bradshaw, P.L. and Bradshaw, G. (2004) *Health Policy for Health Care Professionals*. London: Sage

Health Policy for Health Care Professionals is a contemporary guide to the health service, its origins and current agenda, which focuses on the challenges faced by health service workers in implementing government policy at local level. The book's aim is to help health care professionals make assessments of health policy by giving them an understanding of the ideological basis of the British health care system and the challenges facing the modern National Health Service. It begins with the development of the NHS and its place within the broader context of state welfare provision. The book looks at the options available to governments in formulating policy which responds to health needs. It examines the policies set by recent governments and the feasibility of achieving objectives set by New Labour's *NHS Plan*.

Crinson, I. (2008) *Health Policy: A Critical Perspective*. London: Sage

This book provides a critical assessment of developments in health and health care policy. Primarily focusing on the UK, the chapters cover issues such as the policy-making process, the development of the NHS, health care governance, health promotion and the comparative analysis of health care systems within the EU and US.

Each chapter brings together social and political themes to offer a combination of theory, historical detail and wider social commentary. Case studies illustrate how policy has evolved and developed in recent years, and the implications these changes have for practice. Each chapter includes case studies to illustrate the planning, implementation and assessment of specific policies.

The Joseph Rowntree Foundation **www.jrf.org.uk**

The Joseph Rowntree Foundation (JRF) and Joseph Rowntree Housing Trust (JRHT) are two independent charities that work together to understand the root causes of social problems, identify ways of overcoming them, and show how social needs can be met in practice. JRF is an endowed foundation that funds a large, UK-wide research and development programme. JRHT is a registered housing association, managing around 2 500 homes, and is a registered provider of care services. Their purpose is to **influence** policy and practice by **searching** for evidence and **demonstrating** solutions to improve:

- the circumstances of people experiencing poverty and disadvantage;
- the quality of their homes and communities;
- the nature of the services and support that foster their wellbeing and citizenship.

JRF and JRHT have no political affiliations and work in partnership with all sectors – private, public and voluntary. They aim to present evidence in a balanced, unbiased way and to stimulate debate on current and emerging issues. The work they do includes: looking to reflect the diversity of the UK population, learning from others and operating in a sustainable way – socially, environmentally and economically – finding practical and realistic solutions and focusing on the needs of disadvantaged people.

The website thus contains a plethora of interesting and useful thought-provoking commentaries on health and social care issues.

Chapter 3

The Contemporary Context of Health and Social Care Practice

This chapter covers the following key issues:

- transformation of adult social care services;
- health care modernisation;
- person-centred care;
- personalisation and self-directed support;
- risk and safeguarding.

By the end of this chapter you should be able to:

- discuss the political, economic, social and technological context of change in health and social care practice;
- demonstrate an understanding of personalisation and self-directed support in adult social care practice;
- demonstrate an understanding of person-centred care;
- discuss the importance of informed decision-making and issues of capacity;
- demonstrate an understanding of the notions of risk, vulnerability and professional responsibilities in safeguarding vulnerable individuals;
- consider why these factors influence the ASPIRE care process.

This chapter matches to the following National Occupational Standards and Essential Skills Clusters:

- ESC 1.iii Promotes a professional image;
- ESC 1.iv Shows respect for others;
- ESC 1.v Is able to engage patients/clients and build caring, professional relationships;
- ESC 2.1 Actively involves the patient/client in their assessment and care planning;

- ESC 2.2 Determines patient/client preferences to maximise comfort and dignity;
- ESC 3.1 Takes a person-centred approach to care;
- ESC 11.i Acts within legal frameworks and local policies in relation to the protection of vulnerable adults and children.
- NOS 2.3 Work with individuals, families, carers, groups and communities to enable them to analyze, identify, clarify and express their strengths, expectations and limitations;
- NOS 4.1 Identify the need for legal and procedural intervention;
- NOS 18.1 Review and update your own knowledge of legal, policy and procedural frameworks;
- NOS 21.1 Contribute to policy review and development.

INTRODUCTION

Health and social care is a dynamic area of activity, with constantly changing policies, laws and processes in response to changing health and social care demands and ideas about how best to provide for these. The factors influencing change in health and social care that have been discussed in the previous chapter can be summarised as PEST (political, economic, social and technological) (Businessballs, 2009) and are explained as follows.

- **Political**. This refers to the ideological context, with the emphasis on a needs-led service, rather than service-led provision, with the aim of maximising independence and promoting wellbeing.
- **Economic**. This refers to the rising cost of provision, due to demographic changes and other factors such as globalisation and advances in pharmaceuticals, and the need for more efficient and cost-effective services.
- **Social**. The social model of health and social care (see Chapter 1) is increasingly influential in determining policy. This has been particularly influenced by the disability rights movement, arguing for increased control over services and the determination of need, and has subsequently spread to other service user groups. This has led to a much greater emphasis on empowerment and user-led services, which can be illustrated in the personalisation agenda of adult social care (discussed later).
- **Technological**. The late twentieth and early twenty-first centuries can be categorised by the massive increase in the use of technology

across the whole of society. This manifests in health and social care through the emphasis on high tech care and intensive home care, fundamentally altering the service user journey and the role of hospital and other institutional care. In addition, developments in ICT have far-reaching implications for record keeping in health and social care (see Chapter 6), as well as providing greater independence for service users (see Chapter 8).

The nature of health and social care is transforming to reflect contemporary trends of population growth, demographic changes, and increased public expectations about their needs and how services can be used to address these needs. When the NHS was established in 1948 to manage the illness and disease burden of society (Klein, 2005), hospital-based care was central to the organisation of health care services. It soon became apparent however that this was not meeting the changing health care needs of the population (Jones, 1994). Nettleton (2006) summarises the changes in health and social care as follows:

DISEASE ⟶ HEALTH

HOSPITAL ⟶ COMMUNITY

ACUTE ⟶ CHRONIC

CURE ⟶ PREVENTION

INTERVENTION ⟶ MONITORING

TREATMENT ⟶ CARE

PATIENT ⟶ PERSON

Table 9 Summary of changes in health and social care

There has been a growing mismatch between the health and social care needs of the population and the organisation of health care services throughout the second half of the twentieth century, and transformations in morbidity and mortality, public expectation and the increasing blurring of the boundaries between health and social care have led to a fundamental reorganisation of services in the twenty-first century (DH, 2007b).

Since 1997, there has been a modernisation programme in relation to health and social care services, which has focused on the following key issues:

- the emergence of choice and involvement for service users and carers (person-centred care);
- an emphasis on independence;
- growth in partnership working;
- integrated teams;
- improving specialist services;
- support to carers;
- modernising legislation;
- tackling discrimination and social exclusion;
- commissioning and funding issues.

These key issues are relevant to both adult services and children's services, although the paradigms of care have developed rather differently and have had a direct influence on the care process (ASPIRE).

PERSON-CENTRED CARE

Central to the health and social care reforms under New Labour is the concept of patient/service user care. This involves placing the service user at the centre of the decision-making process and locating the assessment of needs within their own definition of need and within the context of their lives. Person-centred care is central to government reforms in health care (as discussed in Chapter 2), and this has developed through assessment processes (see Chapter 4), service user participation in the planning and intervention phases of care delivery (see Chapters 5 and 6), and the centrality of user and carer evaluations in the quality monitoring process (see Chapter 7). This paradigmatic shift can also be evidenced in the fundamental changes that have taken place in the delivery and funding of health and social care services, through packages of direct payments, personalisation and self-directed support, and the change in focus can be seen across both adult and children's health and social care.

Developments in children's services

There has been a fundamental shift in the way that children's services are provided, with a growing acknowledgement of the need to hear children's voices in relation to health care decisions and protection from risk.

Throughout the twentieth century, there was a change in the way that childhood was viewed in Western societies, with increased respect for children as individuals with rights and choices. This change in societal attitudes was first evident in statute under the 1908 Children Act, which indicated an ideological shift in attitudes to children and policies in relation to children, young people and families and continued throughout the twentieth century, culminating in the Children Act (DH, 1989c) and *Every Child Matters* (DH, 2003c).

Every Child Matters is a framework for practice that identifies the rights of children. Every child has the right to:

- be healthy;
- stay safe;
- enjoy and achieve;
- make a positive contribution;
- achieve economic wellbeing.

The *Every Child Matters* agenda has been further developed through publication of the *Children's Plan* in December 2007 (DH, 2007c). The *Children's Plan* is a ten-year strategy to make England the best place in the world for children and young people to grow up.

Across the spectrum of health and social care, service users and carers are demanding to have their voices heard and children and young people are no exception, as they claim the right to make decisions that impact on their lives. This is illustrated in the following quote from a young person.

> Everyone wants to make decisions for me and it really hurts.
> (Commission for Social Care Inspection, 2007)

Therefore, hearing children and young peoples' voices is central to the policy shift in health and social care provision. However, this raises issues about capacity and whether the young person is able to make decisions concerning their health and social care needs and whether they have the ability to make assessments and judgements about care and interventions.

Gillick Competence or the Fraser Test

Children may not necessarily be seen as having the capacity to consent and the need to safeguard and protect the child from risk outweighs their right to self-determination. With respect to children's competence to consent to treatment, the Gillick Competence test is important. This resulted from a case brought by Mrs Victoria Gillick, a mother of ten children (five boys and five girls), who stated that a doctor would be guilty of encouraging under-age sex if he/she prescribed contraceptives for a child under 16. The claim was considered in the House of Lords, and it was decided that:

> A child who is competent can consent to treatment. However, a parent or the Court where such a refusal would be likely to result in the death or permanent disability of the child may override a refusal of treatment. Then the wishes of the child may be overridden to preserve his or her long-term interests.
>
> (DH, 2001d)

This came to be known as Gillick Competence or the Fraser Test (Lord Fraser was the presiding judge) and has been adopted as the benchmark for professionals to judge the ability of children to provide consent to health and social care treatment in the UK. Similar judgements have been passed in Australia and Canada.

The Gillick Competence test requires professionals to consider the following in making their judgement about the child's ability to consent to treatment.

a) Children under 16 can truly consent to treatment only if they understand its nature, purpose and hazards.
b) To be able to consent, the child should also have an understanding and appreciation of the consequences of:
    (1) The treatment,
    (2) A failure of the treatment,
    (3) Alternative courses of action and
    (4) Inaction.

(DH, 2001d)

The Gillick Competence test focuses on the child's ability to consent not on parental rights or other people's views about rights. There is recognition that it is good practice to involve families of children and 16 and 17 year olds in health care decisions, but also stresses the importance of confidentiality unless there is evidence that this may place the child at risk.

A person over the age of 16 is presumed to have capacity to consent unless there is evidence to the contrary, and they therefore should be treated the same way as competent adults.

Developments in adult health and social care

The shift in the nature of morbidity has altered, with far more people living with long-term conditions, requiring ongoing care and support. Although hospital care remains important within adult health and social care (*National Service Framework for Older People*, (DH, 2001c) – Standard 3: *National Service Framework for Long-Term Conditions*, (DH, 2005b), Quality Standard 4), it is seen as part of a longer and broader stage in the service user's health and social care journey. In addition, the period of hospitalisation has become shorter and more intense, with greater emphasis on community care and the role of the primary health care team. The ageing population and the increased number of people with disabilities and long-term conditions has led to questions about the financial sustainability of service-led provision of care while, at the same time, the notion of the professional expert in health and social care has been contested, with greater demand for person-centred care, reflecting the needs of the individual and their expertise in their understanding and management of care needs.

Two significant policy changes in relation to adult social care are the introduction of the Single Assessment Process (SAP) for older people and the Care Programme Approach in mental health.

The Single Assessment Process

The Single Assessment Process was introduced in 2004 as part of Standard 2 of the *National Service Framework for Older People* (DH, 2001c) and is concerned with making assessment and care planning when working with older people 'person-centred, effective and co-ordinated' (DH, 2002e). This emerged from concerns about inter-agency working and duplication of efforts in relation to information giving and assessments. In addition, there is a focus on assessment processes for protection and safeguarding within the SAP, which raise important issues about multi-disciplinary working (Penhale and Parker, 2008).

The SAP can be seen to mirror the ASPIRE process of care, with stages of assessment, planning, intervention and evaluation, as well as four different levels of assessment, reflecting different levels of need (see Chapter 4).

The stages of SAP:

- Publishing information about services.
- Case finding (seen as optional).
- Completing an assessment.
- Evaluating assessment information.

- Deciding on what help should be offered (including eligibility decisions).
- Care planning.
- Monitoring and reviewing.

The SAP aims to provide a universal assessment tool to cut out the postcode lottery of care in older people's services, provide more continuity of care and a more comprehensive system of care services.

> Wherever you are in England, you will have the right to have your care needs assessed in the same way. And you will have a right to have the same proportion of your care and support costs paid for wherever you live.
>
> You will be able to take your needs assessment with you wherever you go, so wherever you are in England, the assessment of your needs will be the same, enabling you to live the life you want wherever you want.
>
> (DH, 2009d: 53)

The Social Services Inspectorate (1997) found that the most successful assessments of older people were those where a variety of relevant professionals worked together and in collaboration with service users and carers to address service user needs, and the SAP is intended to formalise these arrangements. These issues will be discussed further in Chapters 4 and 5.

The Care Programme Approach (CPA)

The Care Programme Approach was introduced in 1991 as an approach for working with people with complex and enduring mental health problems. The approach focuses on multi-disciplinary work and intensive support for people considered to be 'high risk' and is led by health service agencies (Payne, 2006). CPA was redefined in 2008 so that policy is clearer and more consistent and unnecessary bureaucracy is avoided (DH, 2008a). The CPA focuses on providing high quality care, based on individual assessments of need and addressing the range of needs that the service user identifies through thorough assessment and planning of interventions. Quality measurements are based on reported improvements in service user experiences and outcomes. The CPA can be seen as part of a wider process of whole systems approaches, which were part of the modernisation agenda for mental health practice. Modernisation of mental health services was concerned with the provision of safe and effective care to protect the public, providing a full range of services when needed and working supportively with service users and their families and carers. Individual assessments are fundamental to this modernised approach, as well as providing better care and treatment with 24-hour access to home and hospital services, with a stronger role for primary health care providers. User and carer involvement in decision-making is emphasised as well as the need for accountability through the use of evidence-based practice. The emphasis is on 'whole systems development, which will address the most conspicuous gaps in service provision. We cannot afford to focus on any single aspect of the mental health system and hope that this will provide a solution' (*Mental Health Policy Implementation Guide* (MHPIG) DH, 2002a:3). Elements of a whole systems approach include:

- a range of disciplines is involved in the whole care process;
- complex systems of care are effectively co-ordinated within multi-disciplinary teams;
- good communication between agencies and different elements of the service is essential;
- there is a need for clear leadership and management;
- local service delivery is seen as effective, as local needs can be appropriately addressed;
- user and carer involvement is central to all levels of decision-making;
- professional power is contested, with acknowledgement of different notions of expertise.

The Single Assessment Process and the Care Programme Approach clearly reflect changing practice with service users and carers, and emphasise the importance of person-centred approaches and user and carer involvement in the assessment and planning of services and interventions. In addition, they reflect a change in ideology in relation to power and service delivery, which is also illustrated in developments in the personalisation agenda in adult health and social care services.

PERSONALISATION AND SELF-DIRECTED SUPPORT

Direct payments

Direct payments, personal budgets and self-directed support are part of the government's plans for the personalisation of adult personal care services to address individual needs. This personalisation agenda aims to put the service user in control of the organisation and management of the purchasing of care packages tailored to their individual needs (Stainton and Boyce, 2004).

Direct payments were introduced in the Community Care (Direct Payments) Act 1996 (DH, 1996) for all adults of working age and were extended to older people in 2000. Direct payments can be partly attributed to the campaigns by people with disabilities who actively campaigned for greater control over the services that they wanted and their empowerment through this control.

> Disabled people campaigning for direct payments argue that the resourcing by the state of their effective demand for personal assistants constitutes genuine empowerment through the extension to them of their contractual rights, in contrast to the purely rhetorical empowerment underwritten through procedural rights, where the gatekeepers to care resources remain social workers and health care professionals.
>
> (Morris, 1993, in Ungerson, 1997)

Although the Labour Government has promoted the policy of direct payments, there has been an issue of low take-up, particularly among older people and people with learning disabilities. In an exploration of services for people with learning disabilities, the Department of Health identified that very few people with learning disabilities were in receipt of direct payments and that there was still considerable progress to be made in this area (*Valuing People*, Department of Health White Paper, 2001b,). The Commission for Social Care Inspectorate (now part of the joint CQC with health care) found that, in March 2008, there were 661 000 older people in receipt of community care services and yet only 3 per cent were in receipt of direct payments. Fruin (2000) also points out that there has been significant local variation in the implementation of direct payment schemes by Local Authorities.

In April 2003, regulations came into force that required all Local Authorities to offer direct payments to all people in receipt of community care services and, as the tables below illustrate, there has been a steady increase in the numbers of service users who are in receipt of direct payments in England and Scotland. However, there is still more work that needs to be done in this area and care managers, social workers and health care practitioners are ideally placed to promote direct payments.

Year	Numbers in receipt of direct payments
2005	22 100
2006	32 000
2007	40 600
2008	55 900

Table 10 Take-up of Direct Payments in England (source: Samuel, 2009)

Year	Numbers in receipt of direct payments
2005/6	1 829
2006/7	2 291
2007/8	2 605

Table 11 Take-up of Direct Payments in Scotland (source: Samuel, 2009)

Personal budgets extend direct payments, in that they are the allocation of funding following an assessment of needs that is designed to address those needs. Service users may either take this as a direct payment or they may leave the Local Authority with the responsibility of commissioning services on their behalf, while maintaining the ability to make decisions about how and by whom their care needs will be met.

Individual budgets are an extension of personal payments although they differ from them in that they provide self-directed support through the integration of funding streams, which include adult social care budgets as well as funding from the Supporting People Programme, Disabled Facilities Grant, Independent Living Funds, Access to Work Funds and funding for community equipment services. Close (2009) identifies six ways that individual payments may be managed.

1. Direct payments, which are paid to the individual on a regular basis to directly pay for care and support.
2. Indirect payments to a representative on behalf of the care recipient. This might be a family member or close friend.
3. Indirect payments to a trust, which is a group of individuals who have formed a legally constituted trust, and would usually consist of family members and/or friends of the care recipient.

4. Brokered payments, which are managed by an independent broker, who would normally charge a fee for the service.
5. Individual service funds, where the Local Authority makes regular payments to a service provider in advance of a package of care being delivered. This allows the care provider and care recipient the flexibility to negotiate the design and redesign of care packages.
6. Care managed payments, which are managed on behalf of the care recipient by a social worker or care manager.

The Labour Government signalled its intentions to promote independence and extend individual budgets to all adult service users of community care services through the Green Paper (DH, 2005a) *Independence, Wellbeing and Choice*, in which it stated that services should be based on 'the principle that everyone in society has a positive contribution to make to that society and that they should have a right to control their own lives'. These strategic changes were further developed in the White Paper (DH, 2006a) *Our Health, Our Care, Our Say* and in the 2007 Paper *Putting People First* (DH, 2007b).

At the same time, a similar project of individual budgets, aimed mainly at people with learning disabilities was piloted by MENCAP and the Department of Health's Valuing People Support Team through the In Control Programme, which allocates individual budgets on the basis of self-assessment of need, and enables the service user to purchase the range and mix of services that they feel will best meet their needs.

Activity

Consider how direct payments may impact on the ability of a disabled mother to care for her children and then read the case study below about Sobia.

Case study

Sobia talks about her aspirations as a young South Asian mother of two. She lives in Oldham and has been battling with disability and depression. Prior to In Control, Sobia's support came from conventional Local Authority services that did not meet her requirements. A local agency offered no improvement. The staff showed no knowledge of her cultural needs and religious beliefs.

Sobia said: 'I want to be able to support my children and not be judged because of my disability . . . I am now – and can still carry on being – a good mother to my children'.

Her previous support services had shown no grasp of simple tasks like shopping for certain ingredients and cooking certain meals. She also found that staff did not understand the importance of attending the mosque at regular times for both Sobia and her children. When she heard about In Control, she felt hope for the first time.

Here was a means of support that would respect who she was. Realising that her needs were not being met by the local services, her care manager told her about In Control and its new, simpler approach to the receipt of payments. She also found she could have control over the recruitment of staff from her own cultural background, with additional help from Bridging The Gap. The new support would be so much more flexible.

> I have had a lot of concern with direct payments as regards to the amount of paperwork involved and . . . using the money in the way I wanted to meet my primary needs. In Control, I felt, could provide me with . . . more flexibility and less bureaucracy.

Sobia's depressive condition improved greatly once she adopted this new way of controlling her life.

> I have been able . . . to recruit my own staff and have much more control over the way I am supported, with the shift in services in Oldham to a system of individualised support. I would recommend this approach to anyone who needed support. However, I think it is just as important to have the support of a good care manager and a LINK organisation like Bridging the Gap who helped me with all the practical steps. This made a big difference.

In Control available at **www.in-control.org.uk**

Activity

Visit the In Control website (**www.in-control.org.uk**) and look at a range of case studies.

List the different ways that individual budgets have been used to deliver person-centred care, based on the service user's identification of need.

Following the extension of individual budgets in the 2005 Green Paper, 13 pilot sites were established, and were evaluated in October 2008.

- There was little difference in the average cost of individual budgets and conventional social care support. However, if individual budgets are to be rolled out nationwide, there will need to be significant investments in staff training.
- People who were in receipt of individual budgets were likely to feel more in control of their lives.
- There were variations in the levels of satisfaction experienced by people in receipt of individual budgets, with people with mental health problems and people with physical disabilities expressing the greatest levels of satisfaction and older people expressing the lowest levels of satisfaction.
- A proportion of older people felt that having control over an individual budget for their care placed a greater burden on them.
- Staff had some problems in integrating the different funding streams that are available through individual budgets and found some legislative barriers.

(Samuel, 2009)

Personalisation

Personalisation, including a strategic shift towards early intervention and prevention, will be the cornerstone of public services. This means that every person who receives support, whether provided by statutory services or funded by themselves, will have choice and control over the shape of that support in all care settings.

(DH, 2007b)

The personalisation agenda follows on from Direct Payments, the piloting of Individual Budgets in a number of local authorities and from the pressure from disabled people regarding the provision of care that is controlled and managed by disabled people for disabled people. Inherent within this approach to care are the notions of citizenship and human rights, with respect for individual rights and needs and the promotion of the inclusive society.

> The work on direct payments and individual budgets, alongside that of In Control, are crucial to delivering greater personalisation, choice and improved quality. They are not separate initiatives or fleeting experiments, but fundamental components of a future social care system.
>
> (DH, 2007b)

This future health and social care system is based on the belief that every person has the right to individual living, self-determination and an individual budget for which they are accountable and responsible. This raises issues about mental capacity and the ability to make informed choices, which will be discussed later. It is based on a number of policy imperatives, including user involvement and empowerment (Beresford, 2007) and the concept of inclusivity and valuing people (Walker and Hennessy, 2004), as well as reflecting important theoretical perspectives such as the social model of disability, which has been fundamental in the fight for empowerment and independent living for people with disabilities (see, for example, Swain *et al.*, 1993).

This agenda is aimed at helping people to live their lives in the way that they want, maximising independence through the provision of care and support in consensus with the service user and providing choice and control within all care settings. There are a number of different approaches, although the main approach is

> through the development of a system of self-directed support within which people are offered an upfront allocation of resources – a personal budget (or their own money) – using this flexibly to decide how to achieve their desired outcomes. In addition **person-centred approaches** and **information and advocacy services** are used to ensure that people can gain choice and control whatever their circumstances or type of services used.
>
> (*Personalisation Toolkit*, DH, 2008b)

Personalisation involves a paradigmatic shift in adult social care and provides a new operating system of care, which transfers power from health and social care practitioners to service users and carers, where service users self-assess needs and care and support is tailored to 'fit' the individual rather than to 'fit' the system. The Local Performance Framework drives the system and it is expected that there will be a significant shift towards fundamental system-wide change by March 2011.

There are seven steps involved in personalisation:

1. Setting of a personalised budget based on the service user's assessment of need.
2. Planning the support and care package in consensus with the service user.
3. Agreeing the plan of support and care – what is going to be provided and by whom.
4. Managing the individual budget.
5. Organising the support.
6. Living life as independently as possible.
7. Reviewing and learning and redesigning the package of care and support as necessary.

(Henwood, 2008)

Implications for practitioners in health and social care

This transformation of adult social care services involves a paradigmatic shift in thinking and alters the role of health and social care practitioners, particularly in relation to personal and social care. The personalisation agenda places more emphasis on the advocacy and brokerage role of the practitioner (discussed in more depth in Chapter 4). There is a cultural change, in that rather than providing services and being accountable for the budget, health and social care practitioners and agencies need to trust people to manage their money, although there will be light touch monitoring. This also raises challenges about what we mean by social care and what is appropriate for a person to purchase in their care and support package, which may raise issues about the services that are commissioned and how they are commissioned, as people may move beyond conventional social care arrangements for their care and support. It also raises issues about risk management and safeguarding arrangements (discussed below).

Capacity

The shift towards self-assessment and self-directed support raises important issues about mental capacity and whether the person is able to make an informed decision to assess their needs and plan and manage a package of care. Capacity to make a decision involves having the ability to understand information in relation to that decision, ability to retain that information, the ability to weigh decisions and use information to arrive at a decision and the ability to communicate that decision. The Mental Capacity Act of 2005 is important in establishing the legal parameters for assessing capacity, with the aim of working positively on the basis of working towards capacity and using advocacy to ensure that any decision that is made on behalf of a person deemed not to have the capacity to make a decision is made in their best interests. It should be presumed that adults have the capacity to make their own decisions unless it is proved otherwise. The Act is underpinned by five key principles.

1. A presumption of capacity – every adult has the right to make his or her own decisions and must be assumed to have capacity to do so unless it is proved otherwise.
2. The right for individuals to be supported to make their own decisions – people must be given all appropriate help before anyone concludes that they cannot make their own decisions.
3. That individuals must retain the right to make what might be seen as eccentric or unwise decisions.
4. Best interests – anything done for or on behalf of people without capacity must be in their best interests and
5. Least restrictive intervention – anything done for or on behalf of people without capacity should be the least restrictive of their basic rights and freedoms.

(Department of Health, 2005c)

Case study

Jordan aged 23 suffered a serious head injury as a result of a motorbike accident. Having spent several months in hospital, he has now been discharged home, with intensive involvement from the community rehabilitation team. Jordan is able to feed himself and can bath and dress himself with occasional help with tasks requiring fine motor movement, such as fastening buttons. He is able to communicate his needs, although sometimes his speech can be difficult to understand. He is very forgetful and often cannot remember where he has put something and has difficulty retaining information. His mother is concerned that he continues to smoke.

- How would you assess Jordan's capacity?
- What factors would lead you to think that he may not have capacity to make decisions?
- What factors would you take into consideration when considering Jordan's best interests?

THE RISK SOCIETY

There has also been an increased emphasis on risk and the risk society, with development of services and practices to safeguard vulnerable people in society (Denney, 2005). Ulrich Beck (1992) has been highly influential in the discussion of risk in contemporary societies and has argued that we live in a risk society, where we are constantly faced with risks and decisions about risk taking. For Beck, this is linked to the developments in social welfare in the Western world in the 1960s and 1970s, with an increased emphasis on consumerism and the rights of individuals. According to Beck (1992) and Giddens (1991) in everyday life we are exposed to risks, which are related to:

- environmental change and degradation;
- population growth and migration;
- new patterns of social consumption and lifestyle practices;
- threats of terrorism and illicit criminal activity such as human trafficking and the drugs trade.

Thus, people are constantly exposed to risks and make decisions about risk taking, which involves weighing likely potential dangers against likely potential gains.

Activity

Think about your own life and lifestyle practices.
1. What risks can you identify?
2. Which of these are based on personal choices (for example, lifestyle practices) and which do you see as beyond your control?
3. What are the potential gains in making these choices about risk taking?

Risks and threats are not equally distributed throughout societies, with some individuals facing greater risks through patterns of social organisation and this has led to a growing emphasis on risk and a risk taking approach in health and social care work with vulnerable people (Titterton, 2005).

Vunerable children

Since the 1980s policy and legislation in health and social care has focused on assessing children who may be vulnerable and safeguarding them from risk. In recent years, British child care policy has changed to reflect a central idea that children are potentially vulnerable, and need support and protection, as evidenced in legislation and policy (Children Act 1989 (DH, 1989c); *Every Child Matters* 2003; Children Act 2004 (DH, 2004c)). Following a number of high profile deaths of children (Maria Colwell, Jasmine Beckford, Kimberly Carlisle, Victoria Climbié and Peter Connelly), there has been a growing realisation that children may be abused, neglected, not listened to, not trusted and not believed by adults who should be caring for them and these adults do not always protect children or make decisions that are in their best interests.

The death of Victoria Climbié and the subsequent Laming Report (2003) marked a fundamental shift in the approach to child protection and the need to safeguard children who are vulnerable. Victoria Climbié was an eight year-old girl who died as a result of systematic abuse by her caregivers, her auntie and her auntie's boyfriend, which eventually resulted in her death. The death was widely reported in the media. Both caregivers were charged under the Criminal Justice System and a public inquiry was held to investigate why statutory services of social care, health care and the police service had failed to protect the child. This led to the development of the Children Act (2004) and *Every Child Matters: Change for Children* (2004) following the recommendations made by the Laming Report. The key messages underpinning these policy initiatives are that:

- there is a need to safeguard and promote the welfare of every child;
- the child should be central to endeavours and interventions;
- all agency staff must work together and share communication (see Chapter 5).

Following the death of Peter Connelly in 2007, Lord Laming prepared a second report (DH, 2009e), further emphasising the need for multi-agency working, clear inspection policies and procedures and the central message that safeguarding vulnerable children is everybody's responsibility.

> There is a clear need for a determined focus on improvement of practice in child protection across all the agencies that support children. New ways should be created to share good practice and learn lessons when things go wrong. Within that context there is a need to strengthen the inspection processes of each of the services responsible for the safety of children. Inspection should not be a stand-alone activity. It should not be only an isolated snapshot. It must be accompanied by a robust developmental process aimed at achieving higher standards of service provision.
>
> (*Laming Report*, 2009e: 61)

Vulnerable adults

There have also been significant developments in policies to safeguard vulnerable adults since the late twentieth century, although these differ from the safeguarding policies for children, in that they do not have the same statutory framework. Although there are a number of legislative processes that can be used to protect and safeguard vulnerable adults, there is no single statutory framework. Penhale and Parker (2008) state that the legislation that exists can be seen as a three-stage process:

1. preventing the risk of harm and abuse occurring;
2. targeting 'at risk' individuals, communities and groups;
3. dealing with abuse once it has occurred.

As can be seen from the following table, there is a plethora of legislation that is available to safeguard vulnerable adults. However, the major piece of guidance for health and social care agencies is the *No Secrets* document (DH, 2002b), which is being reviewed in 2009. This provides guidance not statute, although under Section 7 of the Local Authority Social Services Act 1970, Local Authorities (LAs) have a duty to follow the guidance. The guidance also requires LAs to play a lead role in co-ordinating and developing local policies and procedures, although they have no new legal powers. The guidance requires:

- each local authority to have a safeguarding unit;
- local procedures and resources to be in place;
- the Local Authority to be the central point for contact for safeguarding issues;

Legislation	Objective
Offences Against the Person Act 1861.	Criminal acts of violence and abuse can be prosecuted.
Mental Health Act 1983 and 2007.	Protection for people who may be a danger to themselves or other people.
Protection from Harassment Act 1997.	Protection from fear and harassment from the action of others.
National Assistance Act 1948 and NHSCCA (1990).	Responsibility of councils with social service responsibilities to provide accommodation for people 18 + who need care.
Family Law Act 1996.	Protection from others, particularly with respect to domestic violence.
Domestic Violence, Crime and Victims Act 2004.	Common assault is an arrestable offence.
Family Law Act 2005.	Extends availability of orders to people in same sex relationships as well as people who have never cohabited or married.
Sexual Offences Act 2003.	Protects people who are unable to consent to sexual contact.

Table 12 A summary of legislation that may be used to safeguard vulnerable adults (adapted from Penhale and Parker, 2008)

- the Local Authority to establish links with other organisations to co-ordinate responses to adult abuse;
- common approaches to be developed between health and social care agencies to safeguard vulnerable adults.

Although there have been some calls for safeguarding vulnerable adult procedures to be more firmly embedded in statute (DH, 2004f), there is still no single umbrella legislation in this area, and procedure and practice remain largely based on guidance.

Activity

Look at *Every Child Matters* at **www.dcsf.gov.uk/ everychildmatters** and *No Secrets* at **www.dh.gov.uk**

1. What is your professional responsibility in safeguarding vulnerable children and adults?
2. How does this relate to the ASPIRE process of care provision?

Safeguarding vulnerable adults and children is a fundamental principle of current policy and practice and, as such, all health and social care agencies and practitioners have a responsibility to assess risk and invoke safeguarding procedures when necessary. This reflects wider principles of human rights, which are embedded in the Human Rights Act (1998) and government principles that everyone has a positive contribution to make to society and the right to control their own lives.

SUMMARY

This chapter has built on Chapter 2 and further explored the ways in which policy implementation has changed practice and led to a number of changes in the practice of health and social care. These changes include an emphasis on:

- empowering vulnerable people;
- mobilising community resources;
- promoting wellbeing and primary prevention;
- advocacy of integrated services and accountability;
- promoting holistic governance to meet needs of individuals and communities;
- the relation of these changes to the care process (ASPIRE) has been explored throughout, considering the implications for both practitioners and service users of working within a context of person-centred care, personalisation and self-directed support in adult social care practice;
- informed decision-making and the related issue of capacity;
- risk and vulnerability and the professional responsibilities in safeguarding vulnerable individuals.

Reflection	
Identify at least three things that you have learned from this chapter.	1. 2. 3.
How do you plan to use this knowledge within care practice?	1. 2. 3.
How will you evaluate the effectiveness of your plan?	1. 2. 3.
What further knowledge and evidence do you need?	1. 2. 3.

FURTHER READING

Crinson, I. (2008) *Health Policy: A Critical Perspective*. London: Sage

This book provides a critical assessment of developments in health and health care policy. Primarily focusing on the UK, the chapters cover issues such as the policy-making process, the development of the NHS, health care governance, health promotion, and the comparative analysis of health care systems within the EU and USA.

Each chapter brings together social and political themes to offer a combination of theory, historical detail and wider social commentary. Case studies illustrate how policy has evolved and developed in recent years, and the implications these changes have for practice. Each chapter includes case studies to illustrate the planning, implementation and assessment of specific policies.

Nettleton, S. (2006) *The Sociology of Health and Illness*. Cambridge: Polity

This is a well-written, engaging, and theoretically-informed discussion of health sociology in modern Britain. It blends relevant classical and contemporary theories into an explanation of key concepts and issues and provides a lively, balanced, up-to-date introduction to medical sociology. It also discusses issues of interest to health economists, health services researchers, and health care policy-makers.

'Personalisation' web page on the Department of Health website
www.dh.gov.uk/en/SocialCare/Socialcarereform/Personalisation/ DH_079373

This section of the Department of Health website describes the government's approach to personalisation, including a strategic shift towards early intervention and prevention, which will be the cornerstone of public services.

Chapter 4

Assessment

This chapter covers the following key issues:

- the purpose of assessment;
- the nature of assessment in health and social care;
- tools for assessment;
- self-assessment;
- assessment in context;
- the importance of communication skills.

By the end of this chapter you should be able to:

- articulate the reasons and rationale for undertaking assessments in health and social care;
- discuss the difference between subjective and objective approaches to assessment;
- discuss the advantages and limitations of using tools for assessment;
- identify the changing nature of health and social care and the contested notion of the expert in assessment of need;
- discuss the importance of assessing needs within the context of the service user's and carer's lives;
- understand the importance of communication skills within ASPIRE.

This chapter matches to the following National Occupational Standards and Essential Skills Clusters:

- ESC 2.i Actively involves the patient/client in their assessment and care planning;
- ESC 2.ii Determines patient/client preferences to maximise comfort and dignity;
- ESC 6.i Communicates effectively both orally and in writing so that the meaning is always clear;

- ESC 6.ii Uses strategies to enhance communication and removes barriers to effective communication;
- ESC 6.iv Always seeks to confirm understanding;
- ESC 9.i Contributes to the assessment of physical, emotional, psychological, social, cultural and spiritual needs, including risk factors by identifying, recording, sharing and responding to clear indicators and signs;
- ESC 9.vi Recognises indicators of unhealthy lifestyles;
- ESC. 9.xii Collects and interprets data;
- ESC 14.v Communicates with colleagues verbally (face-to-face and by telephone) and in writing and electronically in such a way that the meaning is clear and checks that the communication has been fully understood;
- NOS 3.1 Assess and review the preferred options of individuals, families, carers, groups and communities;
- NOS 3.2 Assess needs, risks and options taking into account legal and other requirements;
- NOS 3.3 Assess and recommend an appropriate course of action for individuals, families, carers, groups and communities;
- NOS 12.1 Identify and assess the nature of risk.

INTRODUCTION

The nature of health and social care practice has changed significantly in the past few years with the modernisation agenda and recent policy and legislative developments (as discussed in the previous chapters). We have seen how the formal system of health and social care developed as a paternalistic service, designed to provide services to address the needs of people at points of vulnerability within their lives. To some extent, this remains true, as health and social care services remain committed to providing for people at times of vulnerability, although there is also a contemporary emphasis on prevention as well as addressing needs. However, there has also been a shift in emphasis from the notion of professionals as experts, fitting people into the services available, towards addressing the needs of individuals as they themselves define them. Also towards working collaboratively with service users and carers as well as within multi-disciplinary teams (MDT) to assess needs, plan the care process and identify appropriate interventions within the available resources.

Our longer-term aim is to bring about a sustained realignment of the whole health and social care system. Far more services will be delivered – safely and effectively – in settings closer to home; people will have real choices in both primary care and social care; and services will be integrated and built round the needs of individuals and not service providers.

(Our Health, Our Care, Our Say, DH, 2006a)

Good assessment is fundamental to the cyclical process of care, and is recognised within contemporary policy principles and imperatives as a key component of interdisciplinary working with all service user groups (see Chapter 5). Key policy developments in relation to both children and adult service users emphasise the centrality of good assessment. (*Modernising Social Services* (DH, 1998a); *Every Child Matters* (DH, 2003c); The Children Act (DH, 2004c); *Our Health, Our Care, Our Say* (DH, 2006a); *Putting People First* (DH, 2007b); *Shaping the Future of Care Together* (DH, 2009f)).

Assessment is the 'foundation for all effective intervention' (Baldwin and Walker, 2005: 36) and is crucial within health and social care practice. If we fail to assess properly, there is a risk of interventions being based on guesswork or chance or of a ritualised approach to the care process (Thompson and Thompson, 2008; Ford and Walsh 1994). Good assessment is essential for the identification of problems as well as setting goals and planning interventions. The Department of Health defines assessment as follows:

> Assessment is about putting together information on a person's needs and circumstances, making sense of that information in order to identify needs, and agreeing what advice, support or treatment to provide.

(DH, 2009f: 20)

Assessment is not simply about gathering information, determining a person's needs or deciding what services will best address their needs, but is an holistic process and determines the planning and intervention stages of the cyclical process. The assessment stage of care is sometimes referred to as like having 'helicopter vision' (Thompson, 2005) as it provides an overview of the person in context. Good assessment is therefore fundamental for good provision of care, as a narrow focus will limit the options for intervention and inaccuracy will lead to inaccurate planning and interventions.

ASSESSING NEED IN HEALTH AND SOCIAL CARE

So what is assessment and how do we go about assessing a person's needs in health and social care? Firstly, we need to ask questions about the purpose of the assessment – what are you trying to achieve and where do we begin? This is an important question, as it helps to determine the outcomes of the assessment as well as establishing the boundaries of the assessment. Secondly, we need to establish what types of information need to be collected and to whom they are relevant. An assessment that focuses on a particular professional theoretical framework may be necessary to establish a particular course of action (for example, protection from risk), but may militate against collaborative working and an empowering approach to working with service users. This leads on to the third question that we need to ask – whose views should be incorporated? There may be times when an objective assessment is required although, in assessing need, policy imperatives emphasise the importance of person-centred assessments and the subjective interpretations of need according to service users and carers. The final question that needs to be asked is about how to make sense of the information to inform planning and intervention, and crucially, how to record the information. The accurate recording of assessment data is imperative for evaluation to take place, as well as for collaborative and partnership working, and this is examined in detail in Chapter 5. Assessment therefore involves a number of activities, which include:

- identification of the problem and sources of information;
- collection of and collation of relevant information;
- assessing the information;
- analysing the information;
- developing a plan of intervention.

Although this might seem quite straightforward, it involves a number of complex decisions and skills on the part of both the practitioner and the service user. For example, a decision needs to be made about whether the assessment is a one-off event or part of an ongoing process. The identification of the area of concern or the problem in context is therefore crucial in determining how the assessment is carried out and feeds into the ASPIRE process. Frameworks such as the Single Assessment Process can help to guide practitioners through the different levels of assessment and theoretical frameworks or models can help to identify factors to be assessed (see below).

Decisions also need to be made about whether the assessment is based on objective identification of needs, which would involve a scientific or objective approach to the assessment, or the subjective identification of need, reflecting the service user-centred approach as discussed in Chapters 1–3. The nature of assessment is also related to the issue of resources and whether the assessment is designed around addressing the needs of the service user or is focused on assessing people for services and allocation of scarce resources (Parry-Jones and Soulsby, 2001). Assessments may also vary in their purpose. As discussed in Chapter 3, there is increasing emphasis on risk and safeguarding in health and social care and assessments may be carried out on a narrow basis to determine the risk that an individual faces (risk assessment). Alternatively a holistic assessment of need may be carried out, which explores need from a collaborative perspective, understanding risk from the service user's perspective alongside the professional assessment of risk, based on theoretical knowledge and evidence.

Assessment in context

An assessment of an individual's needs has to be considered in relation to the psychosocial and environmental context of that person's life. As discussed in Chapter 1, people make sense of health and illness from their own subjective experiences, and so attitudes and beliefs regarding need and addressing need are shaped within the individual, family and community context (Kleinman, 1988). It is therefore important when working from a person-centred perspective to identify and understand the subjective experiences and understandings that the individuals have. However, it is also important to see beyond the need that is presented and identified, to understand how that need has arisen, how it impacts on the individual and the coping strategies that they already have that can be built upon. As stated above, this is clearly located in frameworks such as the Single Assessment Process when working with vulnerable older adults. Similarly, the Department of Health, the Department of Education and Employment and the Home Office have come together to produce a framework of assessment of children in need and their families which 'provides a systematic way of analysing, understanding and recording what is happening to children and young people within their families and the wider context of the community in which they live' (DH, Department for Education and Employment, 2000, p. viii). This framework builds on the duties of assessment of needs set out in Section 17 of the Children Act (1998) and places an obligation on Local Authorities to assess a child where there have been expressed concerns about the child's wellbeing or suspected maltreatment (Section 47 of the Children Act). The framework sets out imperatives for inter-agency work and establishes clarity about the roles of professionals within the assessment process when working with children, young people and families. Within this framework there are a number of principles guiding the assessment.

- It should be child-centred.
- It should be informed by child development theories.
- It should be ecological in approach. This identifies the risks and strengths in the situation and is based on Bronfenbrenner's (1979) ecological system of human development (see Figure 5), which underpins the Framework for Assessment of Children in Need and their Families (see Figure 6).
- It should ensure equality of opportunity.
- It should involve children and family in the process.
- It should build on strengths as well as identifying difficulties.
- It should use an interagency approach.
- Practitioners should see assessment as a continuous process not a single event.
- Assessments should be carried out in tandem with other actions and services.
- Assessments should be grounded in evidence-based knowledge.

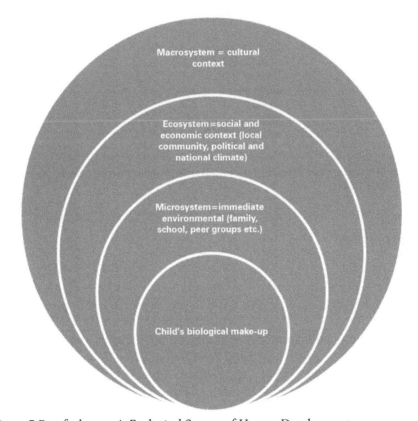

Figure 5 Bronfenbrenner's Ecological System of Human Development

The framework for assessment of children in need and their families provides a systematic approach to assessment and states that each assessment should cover three areas: the development of the child; the capacities of parents and carers to respond to needs; and the impact of wider family and environmental factors. This is known as the assessment triangle and is illustrated in the diagram below.

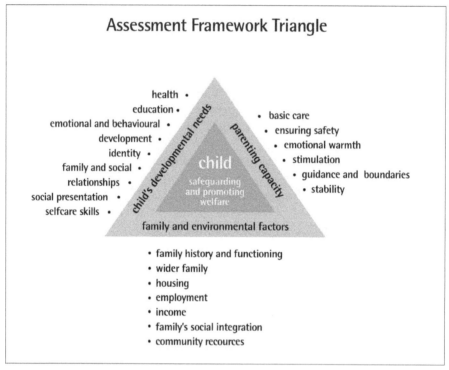

Figure 6 The Assessment Triangle (source: DH, Department for Education and Employment, 2000)

Case study

The class teacher has noticed that Jade aged 9 is frequently late for school, is often dirty and unkempt and has trouble staying awake in lessons. She is falling behind with the work in all key subjects and her performance in English and Maths has deteriorated significantly and is giving cause for concern. Jade can be disruptive in class and, at times, she is quite short-tempered and aggressive with the other pupils in the class. At play times she is fiercely over-protective of her two younger brothers, Aaron and Kyle, who are in lower classes, but also appear to be unkempt, dirty and undernourished. On investigation, it is established that Jade's father has recently been imprisoned for his part in an armed robbery and that her mother is struggling to cope. She is drinking heavily and Jade has taken on the responsibility of not only looking after herself and her two brothers, but also she has been taking care of her mother and trying to manage the household chores, shopping and cooking.

1. Looking at the assessment triangle, identify the factors that will impact on the assessment of Jade's needs and difficulties.

The importance of information in assessment

Assessment is essentially about the collection of data to produce a plan of care and intervention. Data can be derived from the primary sources (the person him/herself), secondary sources (practitioner's observations, data from family and friends) or tertiary sources (other health and social care providers, service user records).

Activity

Look at the case study about Frank on pages 19-20. List the primary, secondary and tertiary sources that you might use to collect data about Frank.

Assessment, then, is an interpersonal activity, which involves a relationship between the practitioner and service user. The data collected may be either objective or subjective, and requires the practitioner to have a number of skills to assess the area or areas of concern.

Activity

Think about an assessment that you have recently carried out or seen carried out by a qualified member of staff.

What skills were needed to undertake the assessment?

Within health and social care, there are a number of ways that data can be collected, involving a range of tools and practitioner skills.

Assessment	Definition	Tools needed	Example
Observation.	Seeing or sensing.	Senses.	Pallor; bruising; withdrawn state.
Interview.	Face-to-face or telephone discussion to discuss a particular issue.	Communication skills. Appropriate environment.	Planned conference. Informal discussion when providing care.
Listening.	Purposefully attending to someone.	Senses. Appropriate environment. Communication skills.	Recognition of underlying concerns.
Consultation.	Using additional resources (e.g. tertiary data sources).	Evidence-based practice. Inter-professional working.	Specialist practitioner to provide additional data.
Inspection.	Close and purposeful observation.	Senses – sight, hearing, touch. Tools such as stethoscope.	More focused than observation – e.g. focused on specific data, such as blood pressure recording.
Palpation.	Use of hands or fingers to examine external surface of the body.	Touch. Vision.	Location of pain. Feeling for a pulse.
Percussion.	Light and sharp tapping on part of the body.	Senses – touch, hearing.	Location of fluid in a cavity – e.g. fluid on the lungs.
Auscultation.	Listening with a stethoscope.	Hearing.	Sounds, such as foetal heart beat.

Table 13 Summary of skills involved in assessment (adapted from Lindberg *et al.*, 1990)

Communication skills

Integral to the assessment process is communication. It could be argued that communication is the most important aspect of the care situation and one that is often overlooked, taken for granted or given little attention by carers. Good communication is a fundamental part of good caring practice and contributes to good quality care as evaluated by care recipients. Even though communication skills have been placed in this assessment chapter it is important to acknowledge that communication is essential to all the steps of the ASPIRE process.

Interpersonal communication is used within any care situation as a planned activity to help individuals and families to prevent or cope with illness or difficult experience and can help people find meaning within the experience (Hayes and Llewellyn, 2008). There is a difference though between thoughtful and thoughtless communication, based on the notion of intention (Heron, 2001). Far from being general chat, purposeful communication, as used by professional carers, demonstrates planning and intention in the development of the interpersonal relationship. It involves guiding, planning and purposefully directing the interaction in order to enable individuals and in some cases empower them to find their own solutions. Thus communication is used as a therapeutic intervention, for example as described by Burnard (1994) in what he called the helping relationship with the client, involving talking, advising and counselling.

Shannon and Weaver (1949) proposed a model of communication that has been used as a basis for explaining communication in a diverse range of fields (Hayes and Llewellyn, 2008). This involves a process where a message is sent via a signal from a source and is received at a destination. Glasper and Quiddington (2009) suggest a communication loop acknowledging that seeing communication as a simple process is fraught with difficulties as inaccuracies can creep in at any time. The complexity of communication within a care encounter is a two-way process and, in the interpersonal relationship, a caring professional will not only transmit a message but will also assess the impact of that message on the receiver, who will give messages back to the sender. Thus health and social care practitioners are both senders and receivers of messages, using more than one strategy and signal to transmit a message. This demonstrates how verbal communication is not simply about words, but includes a whole range of gestures, different sounds, facial expressions and body language.

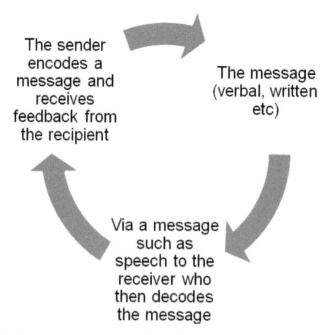

The sender encodes a message and receives feedback from the recipient

The message (verbal, written etc)

Via a message such as speech to the receiver who then decodes the message

Figure 7 The Communication Loop (adapted from Glasper and Quiddington, 2009)

Activity

Think of a practice encounter that you have been involved in.

1. What potential barriers exist for the 'sender' in communicating a 'message'?
2. What potential barriers may exist to prevent the 'receiver' hearing the 'message' as it was intended?

Burnard (1994) summarises the aspects of communication as linguistic aspects (words, phrases, metaphors), paralinguistic aspects (timing, accent, ums and ers, fluency), and non-verbal aspects (eye contact, body language, touch, gesture, etc.).

Activity

Watch an episode of your favourite soap or a film on the television.

1. Make a list of all the metaphors used.
2. Are they effective?
3. Why?
4. What is happening in the script when the characters are using 'ums and ers'?
5. List the situations where touch is used. What effect does it have in those situations?

Key principles to consider when communicating with care recipients can be explored by asking yourself specific questions.

- Can they hear me?
- Will they listen to me?
- Am I giving the 'right' non-verbal signals?
- Am I allowing enough time?
- Am I listening to the person?
- What is the person's story?

Can they hear me?

Always ask the question as to whether the recipient can 'hear' the message. This can relate to physical aspects of hearing – are they hearing-impaired, is there too much background noise, can they understand your spoken language – or they might be so distracted (through anxiety, pain or grief, for example) that they simply cannot listen. It may also be that they cannot understand what you are saying in terms of the use of medical or professional language that they do not recognise. It is important therefore to focus on the person and talk 'with' them rather than 'at' them, therefore adopting a person-centred style rather than a position-focused style (Glasper and Quiddington, 2009).

Will they listen to me?

Is there any reason that the care recipient may disengage? This is also about trust and can depend on developing a rapport with the individual. This is not about becoming 'buddies', but establishing a relationship of trust that enables you to know whether the individual has understood the messages you are trying to convey and is working with you to establish a plan of action as necessary. It is also important that carers consider factors such as appearance. Factors such as how the carer is dressed and their personal hygiene may enable the carer to look professional and may aid the communication process. However, if a person's appearance is scruffy or dirty, this may detract from the communication process.

Am I giving the 'right' non-verbal signals?

Studies have shown that non-verbal behaviours include smiling, service user-directed eye gazing, positive head nodding, leaning forward when talking and touch are essential (Caris-Verhallen *et al.*, 1999). Egan (1990) described the SOLER stance as a useful approach when thinking about non-verbal communication and, in particular, it can aid active listening.

Sit

Open

Lean

Eye

Relaxed

Sit squarely in relation to the client with an **Open** posture. **Lean** slightly forward and use and maintain appropriate **Eye** contact. Try to look **Relaxed**.

Table 14 The SOLER Stance (Egan, 1990)

Am I allowing enough time?

If the individual feels rushed they may feel undervalued and not share important information, so it is useful to communicate to the person that you have enough time or, if you do not, arrange to see the client when you do have time.

Am I listening to the person?

Active listening (Quilter *et al.*, 1993) is an important skill based on being sincerely attentive. It enables the listener to decode the messages they are receiving, demonstrates back to the client that you have understood them and thus establishes good communication, which enables productive dialogue. This can be achieved through reflecting, paraphrasing and summarising, reflecting non-verbal signals and using praise.

What is the person's story?

Communication is not only about the carer's skills of communicating with the care recipients but, importantly, it is also about how the carer enables the individual to communicate their narrative. There is empirical evidence of the benefits of allowing people to talk, which contextualises their suffering within the context of their lives. This helps the carer to understand the situation from the care recipient's perspective as well as identifying resources that they may have to address the problems. Therefore, rather than being an unstructured activity, story telling is a purposeful and planned process, based on sound empirical evidence (Fredrikkson and Lindstrom, 2002).

Negative communications and malignant social psychology

Treachery – using forms of deception in order to distract or manipulate.
Disempowerment – not allowing the person to use the abilities that they do have.
Infantilisation – treating a person in a patronising way.
Intimidation – inducing fear through use of threats or physical power.
Labelling – using a category such as dementia as the main basis for interacting with someone or explaining their behaviour.
Stigmatisation – treating someone as a diseased object or outcast.
Outpacing – providing information, presenting choices, etc. at a rate too fast for the person to understand; putting them under pressure to do things more rapidly than they can manage.
Invalidation – failing to acknowledge the subjective reality of someone's experience.
Banishment – sending a person away or excluding them (psychologically or physically).
Objectification – treating a person as if they were an object with no feelings.
Ignoring – disregarding what somebody is saying or doing
Imposition – forcing a person to do something or denying them the possibility of choice.
Withholding – refusing to give attention or meet an evident need.
Accusation – blaming a person for actions or failures of action that arise from lack of ability to understand.
Disruption – intruding suddenly or disturbingly upon a person's action or reflection.
Mockery – making fun of a person's strange actions or remarks.
Disparagement – telling a person that s/he is incompetent, useless, worthless, etc. Giving messages that are damaging to self-esteem.

Table 15 Summary of negative communications (Kitwood, 1993)

It is very important here to acknowledge that communication can be damaging as well as positive and poor communication can damage self-esteem. Kitwood (1993) explores ways that communication and environment can contribute to the negative experiences of people who have dementia (see Table 15). While Kitwood performed his research and drew his conclusions from work with older people with dementia, the principles can be applied to other areas of care intervention. Negative regard for individuals can reinforce feelings of negative self-worth and self-esteem and thus the way that practitioners communicate is important for wellbeing and person-centred care (see Table 16).

Recognition – acknowledging someone as a unique individual.
Negotiation – consulting about preferences and needs.
Collaboration – working on a shared task, using a person's abilities and strengths.
Play – taking opportunities for spontaneity and self-expression.
Celebration – sharing joyful experiences.
Timalation – sharing sensuous or sensual experiences.
Relaxation – resting either alone or with others.
Validation – accepting the reality and power of someone's experience.
Holding – providing a safe psychological space where vulnerabilities can be expressed.
Facilitation – enabling a person to do what they would not otherwise be able to do.
Creation – creating or offering opportunities for people to offer something to a social setting.
Giving – enabling a person to give to others.

Table 16 Summary of positive ways of communicating

Activity

Reflect on a practice encounter with a service user. Can you identify elements of negative and positive ways of communicating? Reflect on how this knowledge will affect your future practice.

The purpose of assessment

Assessments in health and social care can be undertaken for a number of different reasons including to provide a plan of care, prevention of risk or provision of advice and information to support independence and self-care. Knowing where to begin can be difficult, but identification of purpose will help to provide you with guidance.

Activity

Think about an assignment that you have recently done as part of coursework. How did you identify where to start and how to address the assignment task?

Being faced with an assignment can be a daunting prospect, and it is important to identify the purpose of the assignment to effectively plan how you are going to manage the work, what types of additional information you might require, the timescale for completion of tasks and how you are going to evaluate effectiveness.

The same sort of process is involved in establishing where to begin when undertaking an assessment in health and social care. It may not be possible to assess all needs at once, and the assessment process may need to be staged. If we use the Single Assessment Process as an example (see Appendix 1), we can see that there are different levels of assessment that may not all be carried out when the service user has initial contact with health and social care agencies. The Single Assessment Process was introduced as part of Standard 2 (Person-Centred Care) of the *National Service Framework for Older People* (DH, 2001c) and provides a model for inter-disciplinary assessment of needs. Within the Single Assessment Process there are four types of assessment:

1. **Contact assessment**: this type of assessment is concerned with the identification of the:

- nature of the presenting needs;
- significance of the need for the older person;
- length of time that the need has been experienced;
- potential solutions identified by the older person;

- recent life changes or events which are relevant to the current needs;
- perceptions of family members and carers.

2. **Overview assessment**: this type of assessment is carried out when a more rounded assessment is needed. Within this assessment, there are different domains:

- user's perspective;
- clinical background;
- disease prevention;
- personal care and physical wellbeing;
- senses;
- mental health;
- relationships;
- safety;
- immediate environment and resources.

3. **Specialist assessment**: this type of assessment is carried out when there is a need to explore specific needs in detail and is carried out by the most appropriate qualified person.

4. **Comprehensive assessment**: this is carried out when a specialist assessment indicates all or most of the domains of the SAP are involved, when the service user has a complex set of needs to be addressed. It involves a range of different professionals or teams, although a geriatrician often takes the lead role.

Contact assessment and overview assessment would usually be carried out early in the service user's engagement with health and social care services, so that immediate needs can be established, as well as the service user's and carer's own abilities and strategies to manage any problems or needs. Similarly, if a person presented to the Accident and Emergency Department with some sort of medical crisis, then the purpose of the initial assessment would be to establish immediate goals for intervention. It may be that further assessment would need to take place once the initial crisis has been addressed. (See Appendix 1 for an example of assessment based on the SAP, using the case study about Frank on pages 19-20.)

Characteristics of assessments

Case study

Isabella, aged 36, has been admitted to the Accident and Emergency Department, with acute abdominal pain, haematemesis (vomiting of blood) and shock. Since leaving care at the age of 16, she has spent much of her adult life sleeping rough, or in and out of homeless shelters. She is well known to staff in the Accident and Emergency Department, who are aware that over the years she has become increasingly dependent on alcohol and now drinks at least one bottle of spirits a day.

1. What would you assess Isabella's immediate needs to be?
2. What longer-term needs might you assess?

Exploring the case study above, we can see that there is a need to assess Isabella's level of shock, degree of pain and amount of haematemesis to manage the immediate medical crisis but, once that is resolved, there will be a need to assess her living arrangements, her alcohol consumption and her desire to manage this and any other health problems that have resulted from her living circumstances and lifestyle behaviours.

Although Milner and O'Byrne (2009) discuss linear and holistic models of assessment, it is perhaps more accurate to refer to staged processes of assessment, as this would reflect the different imperatives and purposes of the different levels of holistic assessment.

Activity

Make a list of the ways in which you would assess Isabella's level of shock, degree of pain and amount of haematemesis.

1. What objective measures would you use?
2. What subjective measures would you use?

Looking at the use of both subjective and objective measurements in the process raises a second point about assessment. Is assessment an art or a science?

The science of assessment

A scientific approach is a purposeful approach that is systematic and measures phenomena objectively. The starting point of the scientific approach is to define the problem, before going on to collect data about it, devise and execute a solution and evaluate the solution (Lindberg *et al.*, 1990). Thus a scientific approach to assessment in the above case study would focus on the three problems of shock, pain and haematemesis and look for ways to objectively measure these. Objective measurement is usually carried out by someone other than the person who is experiencing the problem, and therefore places emphasis on the health or social care practitioner's skills and expertise in assessment. There are various tools that can be used to perform an objective assessment. Let us take the example of shock to explore this. Shock occurs because of a lack of circulating blood in the body, which can be caused either by a decrease in the volume of blood (hypovolaemic shock) or by the heart working ineffectively as a pump to distribute the blood (cardiogenic shock). In the case study above, Isabella will be suffering from hypovolaemic shock, as she has lost blood from the haematemesis, which will result in an increase in the pulse rate, as the heart tries harder to pump the required amount of oxygenated blood around the body, while, at the same time, blood pressure will be decreased, as there is less volume of blood. The person may also have a pale appearance and may seem drowsy or even unconscious.

Objective assessment of these symptoms and the level of shock would be achieved through the measurement of pulse rate, using either a machine or the manual method, and the measurement of blood pressure using a sphygmomanometer or electronic method. A health care worker may also observe and record a person's pale appearance, although this measurement is less objective as it incorporates an element of judgement. How do we decide that someone is pale, since we all have unique skin colour and tone?

Similarly, the amount of blood that Isabella is vomiting can be objectively assessed through using a measuring jug and accurately recording the number of millilitres on a fluid balance chart. This becomes more problematic if Isabella is unable to vomit into a receptacle and a judgement is required to determine what constitutes a small, medium or large amount, and then a decision is made on how to communicate this judgement to other members of the health and social care team.

Pain is a subjective experience, but it is possible to employ a systematic approach to the measurement of pain through the use of pain recording charts such as the Smiley Scale, which was devised by the Pain Associates' International Network (see **www.pain-initiative.com/e1833/e5688/ e5885/smiley_engl_eng.pdf**) and asks the person with the pain to identify with one of the five faces that range from broadly smiling to a face screwed up with pain and with tears pouring down the cheeks.

The art of assessment

Assessment of needs is not just a scientific and objective approach, but also relies on subjective interpretations of need. Although knowledge and a credible evidence base should inform practice (see Chapter 6), experiential and tacit knowledge is also important. Experienced practitioners can draw on their previous experiences in similar situations to identify needs and to make sense of data that is presented to them. For example, the practitioners caring for Isabella may rely on tacit knowledge, built on their experience of caring for patients with haematemesis previously, to make judgements on things like, for example, the volume of blood lost when vomited onto the floor, her state of consciousness, and her anticipated experience of discomfort. Experiential knowledge may also help the experienced practitioner to establish the starting point and priorities of assessment, so that both short-term goals and longer-term goals can be addressed. Benner (1984) discusses the transition of nurses from novice to expert. This can be applied to other professionals within health and social care, who will learn and develop skills through reflective practice, development of knowledge and skills and learning from experience.

With the shift in policy and processes from a service-led provision to needs-led provision, with the service users and carers at the centre of assessment and the emphasis on defining need as they themselves identify it, assessment requires a dialogue between practitioner and service users and carers, which in turn requires the practitioner to have good interpersonal and communication skills (see Chapter 6).

Activity

Think about a time when you were assessed. You may think about an exam or your driving test.

1. What did it involve?
2. How did you feel about the process?

TOOLS FOR ASSESSMENT

Throughout health and social care, there are numerous assessment tools that aid the objective assessment of problems and needs. In recent years, there has been a move to develop more systematic tools and assessment forms, in line with government priorities in health and social care, to increase the efficiency and effectiveness of provision, based on a sound evidence base. Some of the better known assessment tools and forms include the Glasgow Coma Scale (see **www.patient.co.uk/doctor/Glasgow-Coma-Scale-(GCS).htm**), which is used where there is suspected neurological damage and includes assessment of vital signs as well as level of consciousness and physical strength. The Waterlow Scale (Waterlow, nd) is a scale devised to assess a service user's risk of getting pressure sores and is used extensively throughout health and social care practice. Within this scale, the practitioner is guided to assess and score a number of social variables and health factors, and then to add up the scores to determine the level of risk (see below).

Build/Weight for Height		Mobility		Special Risks	
Average	0	Fully	0	Tissue malnutrition (e.g. terminal	
Above average	1	Restless/Fidgety	1	cachexia)	8
Obese	2	Apathetic	2	Cardiac failure	5
Below average	3	Restricted	3	Peripheral Vascular Disease	5
		Inert/Traction	4	Anaemia	2
		Chairbound	5	Smoking	1
Continence		**Sex/Age**		**Neurological Deficit**	
Complete/Catheterised	0	Male	1	(e.g. diabetes, MS, CVA, Motor/	
Occasional	1	Female	2	Sensory, Paraplegic)	4-6
Cath/Incontinence of faeces	2	14-19	1		
Doubly incontinent	3	50-64	2		
		65-74	3		
		75-80	4		
		81+	5		
Skin Type/ Visual Risk Areas		**Appetite**		**Major Surgery/Trauma**	
Healthy	0	Average	0	Orthopaedic – below waist,	
Tissue paper	1	Poor	1	spinal	5
Dry	1	NG Tube/Fluids		On operating table – 2 hours	5
Oedematous	1	only/Nil by Mouth/			
Clammy (temp)	1	Anorexic	2		
Discoloured	2				
Broken/Spot	3				
				Medication	
				Steroids, Cytotoxics, High dose	
				anti-inflammatories	4

Score:
10+ indicates a person at risk
15+ indicates a person at high risk
20+ indicates a person at very high risk

Figure 8 The Waterlow Scale (Waterlow, nd)

Activity

1. From the information that you have in the case study above, use the Waterlow Scale to identify whether Isabella has any level of risk from pressure sores.
2. Compare your assessment with that of other students. How much level of agreement is there between your different assessments?
3. How useful is something like the Waterlow Scale for the objective assessment of needs?

While the Waterlow Scale is not a precise scientific measuring tool, as some of the categories are open to different subjective interpretations as well as making assumptions based on age and gender groupings, it does guide practitioners in terms of what they should assess and provides an indication of risk to inform care planning and intervention.

A more holistic assessment tool might guide the practitioner and service user to assess the current situation in the context of wider social, environmental and ecological variables. For example, genograms and life road maps are used as tools to help to identify needs. Genograms are a modified family tree and provide a snapshot of the individual's family and how the service user views it at that particular time (see Figure 9). These are fairly simple to produce but may provide a powerful tool for the exploration of family relationships or identification of life crises that have impacted on the individual.

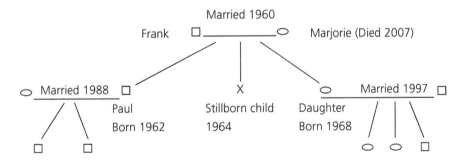

Figure 9 Example of a genogram

> ## Activity
>
> 1. Using the genogram above, identify key points of Frank's life that may have impacted on his current situation (see the case study on pages 19-20).
> 2. Draw your own genogram, identifying key areas that have shaped your current situation.

Models of care and assessment

Models of care also guide practitioners in terms of what they should assess. There are various models in health and social care that place emphasis on different theoretical approaches and provide a framework to guide practice. For example, a number of different models for nursing have developed since the 1960s and 1970s, and these provide nurses with a mental picture to guide their practice. These models can be classified as:

- **Interaction models.** These models place the emphasis on the interaction between individuals and the way in which people behave on the basis of how they interpret a situation or interaction. Meanings and interpretations are context bound and derive from the individual's interactions with others, and the modification of interaction in dealing with situations that are encountered. Not surprisingly, interaction models have been used extensively in mental health nursing, with the emphasis on the importance of interactions between nurse and service user, and including concepts such as communication, role and self-concept. Peplau's model is a good example of this type of model. For Peplau (1952), the focus of nursing was on the therapeutic interpersonal relationship between patient and nurse. Her model is based on humanistic theories and she emphasises the importance of two basic concepts – anxiety and communication, which she views as inter-related (Hayes and Llewellyn, 2008). If communication is seen as threatening in any way, then anxiety results, which is manifested either physically or psychologically. The role of the nurse in Peplau's model is thus tied up in the interpersonal process and the therapeutic relationship. Peplau sees the interpersonal process as having four sequential phases, which help individuals to problem-solve and emotionally mature. These phases are:

  - orientation, where the nurse makes the care recipient aware of the availability of help;

- identification, where the nurse facilitates the expression of feelings;
- exploitation, where the nurse uses communication skills to help the care recipient view problems realistically, and work to reduce the anxiety so that they may personally grow;
- resolution, the final phase, where the care recipient becomes independent and disengages from the interpersonal relationship.

- **Developmental models**. These models focus on stages or processes of development or change to explain the nurse/patient interaction. Self-care, activities of daily living and human needs models all have commonalities in their focus on the human need for life and health. One of the most commonly-used nursing models is the Activities of Daily Living model devised by Roper, Logan and Tierney (2000) that identifies 12 activities that are required for living and health.

Roper, Logan and Tierney's Activities of Daily Living (2000)

- Maintaining a safe environment.
- Communicating.
- Breathing.
- Eating and drinking.
- Eliminating.
- Personal cleansing and dressing.
- Controlling body temperature.
- Mobilising.
- Working and playing.
- Expressing sexuality.
- Sleeping.
- Dying.

While dying may seem a strange activity of daily living, it is incorporated as an important aspect of human existence. This model therefore guides nursing practitioners to important aspects of life and health, which can form a framework for assessment, although the practitioner may need to make a judgement about which parts of the model are relevant to each service user.

- **Systems models**. These models use the general theory of systems to describe the focus of the nursing situation. The service user is regarded as a system within the context of other systems, and thus the models focus on the way that the person interacts with stressors within these systems. For example, Roy's Adaptation Model (Andrews and Roy, 1991) uses systems theory to explore how nurses can help service users to adapt to their stressors and their environment. This model comprises the four domain concepts of person, health, environment and nursing, and involves a six-step nursing process. The person is seen as an open, adaptive system. People use coping skills to deal with 'stressors' and health is seen as the process of being and becoming an integrated and whole person. The goal of nursing is, therefore, to promote adaptation in each of four modes, which are physiological, self-concept, role function and interdependence (social functioning) (Andrews and Roy, 1991).

Roy uses a six-step nursing process:

1. Assessment of behaviour in each of the four modes is assessed as adaptive or ineffective as compared to norms;
2. Assessment of stimuli or the factors that influence behaviour is undertaken;
3. Nursing diagnosis identifies the ineffective behaviours and probable cause;
4. Goal setting involves realistic and attainable goals set in collaboration with the person;
5. Intervention is where the stimuli are addressed, using strategies that are appropriate for the individual's adaptation;
6. Evaluation assesses the degree of change and ineffective behaviours are then reassessed and interventions revised.

Activity

Using Roy's Adaptation Model assess Isabella's needs (see case study on page 117) in each of the four modes (physiological, self-concept, role function and interdependence) and identify possible goals and how to evaluate them.

ASSESSMENT AND SOCIAL WORK PRACTICE

Lloyd and Taylor (1995) have argued that although assessment is fundamental to social work practice, there have been few attempts to construct a systematic theory of social work assessment and the nature of social work assessment can be categorised as follows:

- a problem-solving perspective, which focuses on finding solutions to particular problems;

- a subjective perspective, which is concerned with the subjective experience of the service user;
- a political perspective, which frames the assessment within a structural context and aims to identify the structural factors and power differentials that impact on an individual and their area of concern.

(Howe, 1992)

Assessment of needs can adopt a deficit approach to care, identifying problems and solutions to address these problems. On the other hand, a needs-led assessment identifies problems in context and also identifies normal coping strategies and strengths, and can therefore maximise service user independence (Parry-Jones and Soulsby, 2001). For example, Georgina aged 79 has recently been having increasing mobility problems and has sustained minor injuries from a number of falls in the house and while going to the shops. A deficit model of assessment might see the problem in terms of the mobility and assess Georgina as needing to go into care to protect her from further risk. A needs-led assessment would focus on Georgina's needs and her perspective and her coping strategies. She may feel that she needs adaptations to the house and mobility aids to help her to get about more freely in order to help her to stay independent.

Activity

Go back to the case study about Frank on pages 19-20. Can you identify Frank's needs from a problem-solving and a deficit perspective?

The recovery model that is used in mental health practice is a good example of a theoretical model that is person-centred and adopts a strengths approach to care management (Fawcett and Karban, 2005). Similarly, the theory behind the Single Assessment Process is that the service user and carer should be central to the needs assessment, so that their strengths and preferred ways of coping can be identified (Penhale and Parker, 2008).

Activity

Thinking again about Frank's case study from pages 19-20, identify the strengths that Frank has and how his coping strategies can be utilised to manage his current difficulties.

The objective of assessment is to determine the best available way to help the individual. Assessments should focus positively on what the individual can and cannot do, and could be expected to achieve, taking account of his or her personal and social relationships.

(DH, 1989a, para 3.2.3)

It has also been argued that the concept of anti-oppressive practice underpins social work assessment and is derived from humanistic and social justice perspectives (Milner and O'Byrne, 2009). Social work assessment is concerned with understanding the service user within their environment, which includes their value base as well as their location within a social context, including significant others. Working in partnership with service users is key to anti-oppressive practice and involves a relationship of mutual trust and respect.

A partnership approach can recognise an individual's rights to autonomy, safety, inclusion and having their voice heard without denying power differentials.

(Baldwin and Walker, 2005: 43)

An understanding of power and sources of oppression is central to anti-oppressive practice, in order for the practitioner to understand the structural processes and environmental contexts that impact on the service user experience (see Chapter 8).

Dalrymple and Burke (2006) propose an ethical framework for social work assessment that is based on anti-oppressive practice and includes the following elements:

- assessment involves those being assessed;
- openness and honesty are key to the process;
- assessment involves sharing values and concerns;

- assessment acknowledges the structural context of the area for concern;
- assessment should focus on a critical understanding of the reasons for planned actions and the weighing of alternative courses of action by all those involved;
- assessment incorporates the different perspectives of all those who are involved.

Activity

Consider the following quote:

> Nothing quite prepared me for the shock of entering residential care. Most of the staff are incredibly patient and kind – and I appreciate their help – but it is the constant bustle and ringing of bells from which one cannot escape . . . and the limited choice about food, activities or even companionship, which I find so hard to take. Then I am not allowed to do anything considered the least bit risky, one understands it is to keep one safe . . . but it's pretty galling at my age, after a life of independence, to find oneself so powerless and constrained.
>
> (cited in McClymont, 1999)

1. What structural factors might impact on this lady's experience of residential care?
2. How would an understanding of how structural factors impact on the lady help you to assess her needs?

Social work assessment is therefore concerned with understanding people within their social context and is based on a relationship involving trust and mutual respect. An understanding of power and sources of oppression can help the social worker to understand the area of need within the structural context (see Chapter 8) and assessment is based on the notion of partnership and collaboration. Parker (2007) proposes a relationship-based reflective model of assessment, which involves the following stages.

Stage 1 – A shared and transparent understanding of provisional involvement.

Stage 2 – A collaborative construction of concerns.

Stage 3 – A mutually-determined analysis.

Stage 4 – A collaborative strategy for intervention.

The social worker will work in partnership with the service user to identify the area of concern, assess the relevant information and determine the appropriate map or model as a basis for intervention. However, social workers and health care professionals also have an important role in safeguarding vulnerable people and therefore assessment may also be concerned with assessing people's level of risk. Penhale and Parker (2008) identify three overlapping areas of assessment that a social worker may be involved with.

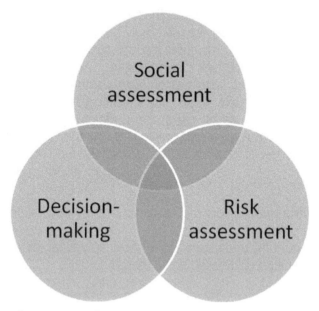

Figure 10 Overlapping areas of social work assessment (source: Penhale and Parker, 2008)

SERVICE USER INVOLVEMENT IN THE ASSESSMENT PROCESS

Neumann (1995) uses a developmental approach to describe the nursing situation and to provide guidance for nursing assessment but, in contrast to Roper, Logan and Tierney's rather rigid model, she proposes the use of six broad questions to gain information from the service user.

1. What do you consider to be your major problem, difficulty or area of concern?

2. How has this affected your usual pattern of living or lifestyle?
3. Have you ever experienced a similar problem before? If so, what was that problem and how did you handle it? Was your handling of the problem successful?
4. What do you anticipate for yourself in the future as a consequence of your present situation?
5. What are you doing and what can you do to help yourself?
6. What do you expect care givers, family, friends and others to do for you?

Although this model was developed for nursing practice, these questions are very general and could be used by any health and social care practitioner to assess an individual's needs and strengths. These questions are also useful as they acknowledge the role of the service user and carers in the caring process and assess service users' own perceptions of their needs and strengths and coping mechanisms. This fits in with contemporary government priorities for care provision, which is person-centred and individualised, as well as reflecting contemporary theoretical approaches to care delivery, such as holistic care and personalised care and the underpinning theory of the Single Assessment Process.

Service users' and carers' own assessment of needs and priorities has become increasingly important in health and social care since the 1990s, and a number of self-assessment tools have developed that place the focus firmly on the individual's interpretation and perception of their needs and acknowledges the subjective nature of assessment.

Self-assessment

The shift in emphasis from health and social care practitioners as experts in the assessment and management of needs to a more person-centred approach, with service users and carers at the centre of the process of assessment, has led to an increase in the use of self-assessment tools in health and social care (Milner and O'Byrne, 2009). These tools can be used by the service user and/or carer in isolation, or can be used as part of a holistic assessment in conjunction with health and social care practitioners. The General Health Questionnaire (available at **www.gp-training.net/protocol/docs/ghq.doc**) is a good example of a self-assessment tool. It asks the individual to rate their own health status using a rating scale to determine how they are feeling in a number of psychological and physical domains that incorporate comparisons with their normal experience. The PHQ-9 assessment tool is a self-administered questionnaire (available at **www.patient.co.uk/doctor/Patient-Health-Questionnaire-)PHQ-9).htm**), used within the community to assess an individual's psychological problems. Self-assessment is therefore important for establishing current needs and problems within the wider context of the individual's life and experiences and for identifying needs as they themselves see them, which can also help to identify strengths and coping mechanisms so that interventions can be tailored to those individual needs. Self-assessment has been particularly associated with the increase in the use of direct payments within a personalisation context (see Chapter 3).

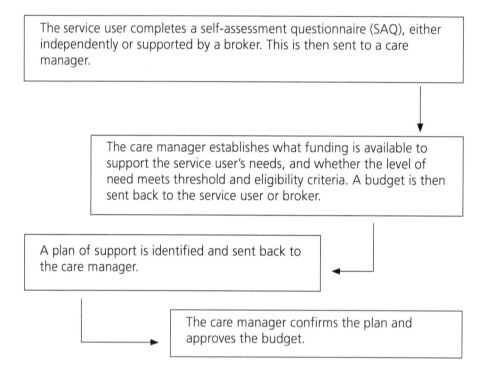

Figure 11 A model to demonstrate the relationship between self-assessment and direct payments (adapted from Milner and O'Byrne, 2009)

As previously stated, assessment is key to processes of care and intervention and the current policy focus is on needs-led assessment, with the service user at the centre of the process. However, Parry-Jones and Soulsby (2001) have identified difficulties in pursuing a model of needs-led assessment. These are related to problems of identifying need due to its conceptual complexity (see Chapter 1), a historical focus on assessing people for services and the lack of a common framework for assessing needs across professional boundaries. The Department of

Health (2009d) has proposed a Common Assessment Framework in adult social care, which aims to provide a better service for the users of health and social care, based on person-centred assessment of needs and care planning. In addition, the proposals set out a strategy for improving the efficiency of health and social care systems through the development of shared electronic assessment tools and records to facilitate safe and timely exchange of information between providers. The focus is on redesigning local structures and systems to facilitate a more co-ordinated approach to the assessment and planning of care. The broad aims of the Common Assessment Framework are to:

- deliver a person-centred approach to assessment (self-assessment) and support and care planning;
- facilitate better identification of the needs of people with complex longer-term support needs (including carers with support needs); and
- underpin seamless service delivery between the NHS and social care by improving integrated multi-disciplinary working.

(DH, 2009d)

SUMMARY

This chapter has focused on the assessment stage of the process of care (ASPIRE). Building on Chapters 1 to 3, which set the historical and policy context, it has explored the contemporary nature of assessment at the beginning of the twenty-first century. The nature of assessment and the essential nature of communication and other skills within the ASPIRE process were discussed. By examining the purpose of assessment, different approaches and tools of assessment and the contemporary focus on self-assessment, the student of health and social care will be able to articulate the reasons and rationale for undertaking assessments in health and social care. Subjective and objective approaches to assessment have been discussed and the benefits of each examined. Tools for assessment have also been identified and their benefits discussed within the changing nature of health and social care and the contested notion of the expert in assessment of need when considering the context of the service user's and carer's lives.

Reflection	
Identify at least three things that you have learned from this chapter.	1. 2. 3.
How do you plan to use this knowledge within care practice?	1. 2. 3.
How will you evaluate the effectiveness of your plan?	1. 2. 3.
What further knowledge and evidence do you need?	1. 2. 3.

FURTHER READING

Hogston, R. and Marjoram, B. (2007) *Foundations of Nursing Practice: Leading the Way*. Basingstoke: Palgrave Macmillan

As the title suggests, this book lays down a broad base of knowledge, covering the physical and psychological sides of nursing care. It is clearly written and supported by both simple illustrations and activities. Each chapter has introductions, summaries, tests, generic case studies as well as useful references and further reading sections. It covers the elements of the ASPIRE process as applied to nursing care.

Milner, J. and O'Bryne, P. (2009) *Assessment in Social Work*. London: Palgrave Macmillan

This book describes assessment as a crucial social work task giving structured, practical guidance on how to approach this vital professional skill. In a clear and accessible style, the authors provide the theory behind assessment as well as helpful practice examples.

At the heart of this book is a set of theoretical maps to guide social workers' thinking and decision-making when undertaking assessment. It gives insights into the kind of high-quality collaborative assessment that is most likely to lead to effective interventions, chapters that discuss the specific challenges of assessment in children's and adult services, careful analysis of the latest legislation and government guidance and engaging features such as case studies, questions to challenge your perceptions, and thinking points to make you consider your own experience in the workplace.

Penhale, B. and Parker, J. (2008) *Working with Vulnerable Adults* (*Social Work Skills*). London: Routledge

Working with Vulnerable Adults provides an understanding of current practice in social and health care, examining abuse of vulnerable adults and the ways in which social policy, welfare services and practitioners may help. It provides an understanding of current professional practice in social and health care, examining abuse of vulnerable adults and the ways in which social policy, welfare services and practitioners may compound or alleviate vulnerability.

Working with Vulnerable Adults develops a sound basis for understanding issues of risk, vulnerability and protection and investigates how agency policies and procedures may, often unintentionally, lead to the voice of service users being marginalised or unheard. The book draws on recent and established research about the protection of vulnerable adults. Much contemporary social and health care practice with adults is concerned with issues of risk and protection.

Chapter 5

Planning

This chapter covers the following key issues:

- the nature of planning care and support;
- goal setting and SMART objectives;
- partnership working within the multi-disciplinary team;
- collaborative working with service users and carers;
- the importance of keeping accurate written records and confidentiality;
- the financial aspects of care planning.

By the end of this chapter you should be able to:

- discuss the importance of the planning phase of the care process;
- articulate the practitioner's role in working in partnership with other health and social care practitioners;
- discuss the nature of working in collaboration.

This chapter matches to the following National Occupational Standards and Essential Skills Clusters:

- ESC 2.i Actively involves the patient/client in their assessment and care planning;
- ESC 2.iv Supports patient/client to identify their goals;
- ESC 9. Make a holistic and systematic assessment of their needs and develop a comprehensive plan of nursing care that is in their best interests and which promotes their health and wellbeing and minimises the risk of harm;
- ESC 7.ii Protects and treats information as confidential except when sharing information is required for the purposes of safeguarding and/or public protection;
- ESC 7.ii Apply the principles of data protection;

- ESC 9.iii Contributes to the planning of safe and effective care by recording and sharing information based on the assessment.
- NOS 4.3 Plan and implement action to meet the immediate needs and circumstances;
- NOS 6.1 Negotiate the provision to be included in plans;
- NOS 6.2 Identify content and actions and draft plans;
- NOS 6.5 Renegotiate and revise plans to meet changing needs and circumstances;
- NOS 7.2 Work with individuals, families, carers, groups, communities and others to initiate and sustain support networks;
- NOS 16.1 Maintain accurate, complete, accessible and up-to-date records and reports;
- NOS 17.1 Develop and maintain effective working relationships.

INTRODUCTION

Although assessment is the cornerstone of good quality care, planning of appropriate interventions is also fundamental to the care process. Care planning involves the notion of partnership working, collaboration and joined-up thinking. Statutory frameworks and guidance have emphasised partnership and collaborative working since the inception of the modernisation framework for health and social care services in 1998 (Department of Health, 1997a and Department of Health, 1998a). Professional codes of practice also emphasise the centrality of partnership working in good quality care. For example, the National Occupational Standard Key Role 2 for Social Work Practice requires social workers to 'Plan, carry out, review and evaluate social work practice, with individuals, families, carers, groups, communities and other professionals' (GSCC, 2002). Also, as stated in the NMC (2007) Essential Skill Cluster – The Organisational Aspects of Care, for entry on to the register nurses must be able to:

> Make a holistic and systematic assessment of their [patients'] needs and develop a comprehensive plan of nursing care that is in their best interests and which promotes their health and well-being and minimises the risk of harm.
>
> (NMC, 2007)

WHAT IS INVOLVED IN THE PLANNING OF CARE AND SUPPORT?

The planning phase of the care process involves the development of strategies to reduce, minimise or address the problem or need that was identified in the assessment phase of the process. Iyer *et al.* (1986) suggest that this consists of four stages.

1. Setting priorities.
2. Developing outcomes.
3. Developing orders (measures or interventions).
4. Documentation.

These stages of planning are important in all health and social care encounters but, in managing the care of someone with complex needs and/or a long-term condition, it is particularly important to identify the priorities of need and support and to develop realistic outcomes, which can be effectively evaluated. Just as assessment is an ongoing process, so the planning phase involves a staged and ongoing systematic process. The single assessment process discussed in Chapter 3 is one tool for determining the layers of assessment, planning and intervention that an individual may require.

Care plans

Care plans relate to the organisation of the care that is to be given to an individual client. It is an essential part of the care journey as described within nursing or social care process models (see Chapter 4). Care plans are used to determine the care given to an individual.

The Framework for the Assessment of Children in Need and their Families (Department of Health, Department for Education and Employment, Home Office, 2000) identifies the following key elements that should be included in a plan of care:

- objectives of the plan;
- what services will be provided and by whom;
- the timing and the nature of contact between professionals and families;
- the purpose of services and contact;
- the commitments to be met by the family;

- the commitments to be met by professionals, including attending to matters of diversity and equal opportunities;
- specification of those parts of the plan which can be renegotiated and those which cannot;
- what needs to change and what goals need to be achieved;
- what is unacceptable care;
- what sanctions will be used if the child is placed in danger;
- what preparation and support children and adults will receive if they appear in court as a witness in criminal proceedings.

While some of these elements are specific to work with children and the safeguarding of vulnerable children, many of them can be related to care planning more widely within health and social care.

Goal setting

Goal setting is an important part of the planning process, and involves predictions about what the care recipient hopes to achieve through the planned interventions. Goals should aim to develop an individual's strengths so that they feel in control of the situation and can share in the problem-solving approach to care. Goals are often written in behavioural terms and should be person-centred to address individual needs. They should also state who expects to attain the result. It is also important when setting goals that the goals are measurable and achievable, and have specific criteria stated to measure the outcome of the planned intervention. The establishment of goals that are measurable enables care to be evaluated and then improved upon (Hambridge and McEwing, 2009).

SMART objectives

SMART objectives are useful when setting goals. This means that goals should be:

Specific;

Measurable;

Achievable;

Realistic;

Time-bound.

Activity

In Chapter 1 we met Frank. Since the death of his wife Frank has been feeling very lethargic and tired, and although generally he has managed to cook for himself, he has become increasingly reliant on ready meals and take-aways. When his daughter visited, she noticed that Frank looked tired and was unkempt and withdrawn. The garden was overgrown and when she asked Frank about the British Legion, he told her that he had not been for a few weeks.

1. Imagine you are the social care worker who has been assigned to Frank's case. What SMART plan can you put into place to address either his nutritional or social needs?

As a guide you may want to consider the following health-related SMART plan investigating the lethargy. The GP's plan is:

Specific – for the specific problem of lethargy his GP investigated Frank for anaemia.

Measureable – there are specific measures that would indicate anaemia as investigated through blood sampling.

Achievable – this test is available on the NHS.

Realistic – Frank agreed to have the blood test and this was undertaken and anaemia can be easily treated or further investigated to identify the cause.

Time-bound – the results would be available within 24 hours.

See Appendix 2 for an example of a nursing care plan to address Frank's needs. See Appendix 3 for an example of a social care plan to address Frank's needs.

MACROS criteria

Another way of setting goals is to ensure that they conform to the MACROS criteria (Hogston, 2007). These are goals that are Measurable (and observable so that the outcome can be evaluated), Achievable and time-limited, Client-centred, Realistic, Outcome written and Short.

Some needs are complex and may require the development of a number of SMART or MACROS objectives, with short, medium-term and long-term goals. This is what is meant by being realistic. Too ambitious a goal can be demoralising, as the individual is unable to see how they can achieve that goal.

Question: What is the best way to eat an elephant?

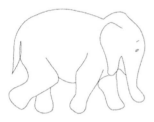

Answer: In small pieces.

The analogy here is that the idea of eating a whole elephant is overwhelming and can outface even the heartiest of eaters. Breaking the elephant down into small pieces and planning to eat it over a long period of time can help to make the task seem more achievable.

Case study

Consider the following case study:

Stuart is now aged 26 and weighs 32 stone. He has been overweight since early childhood and hated PE and games at school as he always felt very self-conscious about his body and quickly got out of breath on exertion, making it difficult to perform in team sports and competitive games. Stuart has therefore got used to leading a sedentary lifestyle and has used food as a way of comforting himself as he has become increasingly lonely and socially isolated. He has now admitted that he needs to lose weight in order to not only feel that he can participate more actively in society, but also prevent further health damage and premature mortality.

1. Using SMART or MACROS objectives, devise a plan of care to help Stuart to achieve his long-term goal of losing half his body weight.

Problem-solving and decision-making

Care planning is based on a process of decision-making and integral to this is the ability to solve problems as faced within the care situation. There are many theoretical approaches to problem-solving and decision-making but all must come with a health warning in that both problems and their solutions can be defined by a myriad of variables and the outcome can be dependent on an individual care recipient's personal choice, one they may be reluctant to share with the caregiver.

Problem-solving models

There are a number of problem-solving models that essentially lead the individual through a process, which attempts to improve decision-making. These include a traditional problem-solving seven-step model:

1. identify the problem;
2. gather data to analyse the causes and consequences of the problem;
3. explore alternative approaches;
4. evaluate the alternatives;
5. select the appropriate solution;
6. implement the appropriate solution;
7. evaluate the results.

In this model the decision is made at step 5.

A second model to improve decision-making is the managerially-based model proposed by Marquis and Huston (2008, p.26), which has the following stages:

1. set objectives;
2. search for alternatives;

3. evaluate alternatives;
4. choose;
5. implement;
6. follow up and control.

In this model the decision is made at step 4.

Common problems with these models lie in the time it can take to fully implement them. Often individuals may try to make decisions without being completely clear about the goals and they can fail because decisions have to be made using available knowledge and information and so it is essential that both the care giver and care recipient have accurate information. It is also common for problem-solvers to be limited in their generation of alternative solutions and so the generation of choices is important.

It is also important to think logically during the process. Dangers arise from overgeneralising and assuming consequences (without evidence). It can also be difficult sometimes to make a choice and act decisively. A consequence of recognising many alternatives is that the decision-maker may be paralysed by choice.

The impact of individual variables

Individual decisions are based on the individual's value system. Regardless of how objective the criteria are, value judgements will always play a part (Marquis and Huston, 2008). Think back, for example, to Stuart in the case study above. Both he and you as the practitioner know he has to lose weight, but his need for the comfort from the food he eats is a greater need for him – it takes a skilled and imaginative professional to come up with a plan that addresses Stuart's needs in a holistic and successful way, which both addresses his need to lose weight and his need for comfort – a need which means an alternative to food is found. Value judgements can be referred to as intuition based on past experiences and professionalism but it is essential to think carefully about the decisions made and justify them according to objective criteria. Developing self-awareness and reflective practice is an important element in problem-solving outcomes.

There are therefore a number of critical elements in problem-solving and decision-making that should always be considered.

• It is essential that decisions have a clear objective.

- Decisions are based on knowledge and so the acquisition of knowledge and information is a clear and important need (for both care professionals and clients).
- As problem-solvers gather information it must be recognised that preference is not mistaken for fact. This is why it is so important that many alternatives are generated in the decision-making process.

Types of decision

It is true to say however that all types of decisions are not the same. Marquis and Huston (2008) defined three types of decision as Routine, Urgent and Considered, arguing that each of these takes a different approach and skill. A routine decision is one that usually does not cause difficulty or disagreement, an urgent decision has an immediate and informed response, and considered decisions are often the most difficult with input from a number of different people, each of whom may be affected by the decision made and who have the expectation, if not the right, to be involved.

Activity

Refer back to the case study concerning Stuart on page 139. Stuart needed to make a number of decisions regarding his future.

1. What type of decision has Stuart already made by deciding to lose weight: routine, urgent or considered?

2. Other decisions made by Stuart may include:

- what his goal will be (weight or physical goal)?
- who will he go to, to seek help in planning a safe and healthy weight loss regime?
- what type of exercise activity can he embark on immediately?
- what type of exercise regime will he build up to and take on long-term?
- how he will plan and undertake his food shopping to avoid buying unhealthy options?

Are these decisions routine, urgent or considered?

3. Who needs to be involved in the decision-making process for each of these decisions?

Collaborative decision-making

Considered decisions within a care situation will normally entail shared or collaborative decision-making and there are a number of steps that must be followed when working in this way. It is essential to consider the context of the service user/client and the context of the health or social care practitioner, the context of the main caregiver (if appropriate)

A single care plan should be developed containing the following information:

- Summary of assessed needs indicating the intensity, instability, predictability and complexity of problems, the associated risks to independence and the potential for rehabilitation.

- Notes on whether or not the service user has agreed the care plan and a reason where not possible.

- The objectives of giving help and anticipated outcome for the service user.

- Summary of how services will impact upon the assessed needs and risks.

- The part the user will play in addressing needs, including their strengths and abilities.

- Details on managing risk. Note any risk accepted by the user.

- Details of what carers are willing to do and related needs and support.

- Description of the level and frequency of the help to be given stating which agency will supply what.

- Nursing plan (integrated and not attached) if any is required.

- Level of registered nurse care contribution for nursing home admissions.

- Name and contact number of care plan co-ordinator.

- Emergency/alternative contact number and a contingency plan if matters go wrong.

- Monitoring arrangements and a review date.

(DH, 2002e)

Table 17 Criteria for the contents of a care plan according to Single Assessment Process guidance

and the context of the situation (Oko, 2008). This will be enabled if the following steps are taken:

- develop a partnership;
- review the service user's preferences for information;
- establish the service user's preference for their role in decision-making;
- ascertain the service user's ideas;
- identify choices;
- present evidence;
- negotiate a decision;
- agree an action plan.

(Towle and Godolphin, 1999)

The Single Assessment Process is a tool for collaborative decision-making in the assessment and planning of care needs (see Table 17). The Department of Health has set out the criteria for the contents of a care plan according to Single Assessment Process guidance (DH, 2002e).

Decision-making tools

It is also possible to adopt a decision-making tool to aid the process (Marquis and Huston, 2008). Decision grids and decision trees are good examples of these tools.

Decision grids

Decision grids are useful as they allow the visual comparison of a number of alternatives against any criteria. The criteria can be anything of relevance like, for example, the cost of an intervention, carer preferences, workforce availability, etc.

	Criteria 1	Criteria 2	Criteria 3	Etc ...
Alternative 1				
Alternative 2				
Alternative 3				
Etc ...				

Table 18 An example of a decision grid

Activity

Think about a decision that you have made recently like, for example, which course to study, or holiday to book, or even something as simple as what to have for your tea tonight.

1. Construct a decision grid to examine your alternatives against criteria which you yourself have set. For example, one of the criteria for a holiday may be cost.

Decision trees

Decision trees demonstrate the decision-making process by illustrating the possible decisions and outcomes of those decisions (Shu-Mei, 2005). Essentially, they allow visualisation of different outcomes and enable the processing of information by trying to illustrate the logical development of a decision and its alternatives and outcomes. They are, however, dependent on the problem-solver being able to both identify alternatives and hypothesise different outcomes and their probabilities.

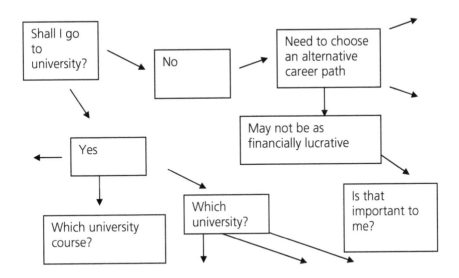

Figure 12 An example of a decision tree

Activity

1. Look at the decision tree in Figure 12. Consider which decisions may be added to the decision tree, especially where there are extra arrows.
2. Do you have an important decision coming up in your life? Try writing a decision tree to help you decide on your options and inform your decision.

Ethical decision-making

Finally, it is always important to take time to consider our own personal values and the impact they may have on practice. This is as important when considering the decisions we make as at any other time in the care relationship. This is dependent on what we as individuals view as the nature and purpose of the caring relationship, our consideration of the nature of ethics within the caring relationship and the components of ethical decision-making.

By considering the ethics of a relationship or a decision we are acknowledging that there is a moral code that underpins practice, based on 'the primary principle of obligation embodied in the concepts of service to people and respect for human life' (Carper, 1978, p.17). In ambiguous situations it may be difficult to predict the consequences of one's actions and the moral content of making difficult personal choices, determining what is good and bad or what ought to be done in a situation, must be considered. In addition, there may be conflicts in the delivery of health and social care, and the ethical dimension of knowing helps to understand and resolve some of these dilemmas. Caring as an ethical foundation for health and social care practitioners should therefore be seen as a moral stance; it is about protection, enhancement and preservation of human dignity (Watson, 1985). Decision-making must therefore reflect the four ethical principles:

- **autonomy** – the right of a person to make their own decisions and direct their life;
- **beneficence** – the responsibility of doing good and so providing benefit or beneficial treatment/care to the person;
- **non-maleficence** – the responsibility of avoiding harm to the person;
- **justice** – the responsibility to be equitable and fair in the way we treat others.

When making decisions in the caring relationship consideration must therefore be given to the following factors.

- The importance of duty or rights in the decision-making process. Whether practitioners in health and social care, for example, have a moral obligation to act in a certain way.
- Whether there are any absolute or fixed principles that guide behaviour. These could be as ethical principles such as 'above all do no harm' but can also be seen in professional codes such as the *Nursing and Midwifery Council Code* (2008) and National Occupational Standards for Social Work.
- The principle of universalism and consistency in decision-making, which can be argued to reflect the principle of utility – the need to achieve the greatest good for the greatest number – and also the principle of justice, which is about equity and could relate to issues such as distribution of services and resources.
- The issues of dignity and worth, welfare or wellbeing and social justice (Banks, 2006).

Activity

Refer again to the case study about Stuart on page 139. Stuart has embarked on his weight loss regime, visiting the Practice Nurse for help and advice. After an initial weight loss of 6 kg the Practice Nurse notices that Stuart has stopped losing weight and, although he keeps coming to see her, he seems to be more interested in chatting about her social life. The Practice Nurse realises that he has stopped following the eating plan they had agreed and notices that he is getting the bus to the surgery when he had agreed to walk as part of his exercise plan. She realises that it is very important that Stuart maintains his weight loss plan but she is very busy and she cannot afford the time to see him weekly if he is not putting in the 'effort' to lose weight.

1. Using a decision tree or a decision grid to explore the outcomes, and referring to the ethical framework above, try to decide what she should do.

Partnership working

All health and social care professionals are now encouraged to work 'in partnership' with other health and social care practitioners and this is embodied in policy frameworks and legislative processes, as well as professional codes of conduct (*Every Child Matters*, DH, 2003c; *Our Health, Our Care, Our Say*, DH, 2006a) (see Chapters 2 and 3). Health and social care professionals are now trained in 'inter-professional learning' but also in terms of seeing working with clients as a type of partnership.

What is partnership?

Literally, working in partnership means working with other people (Thompson and Thompson, 2008). However, this needs to be explored further as, for practitioners in health and social care, it is impossible not to work with other people in the daily working environment. In the context of contemporary health and social care, working in partnership involves working with other health and social care professionals in the multi-disciplinary team, as well as with service users and carers. Collaborative working involves moving away from traditional elitist models of practice based on professional power and expertise, and working collaboratively with service users and carers to identify the problems that need to be addressed and the best way to address them.

Collaboration and user involvement in care planning is crucial to person-centred and individualised care, and needs to focus on the needs and strengths of the individual. The notion of user consultation and involvement is highlighted in the inquiry into the death of Victoria Climbié (*Laming Report*, DH and Home Office, 2003), which identified the need to consult with the child and carers in developing a plan of action (Recommendation 25). Similarly, government guidance in relation to care planning for adult care recipients focuses on the notion of collaboration and consultation with users and carers and the individualisation of the care plan.

> Care planning should be responsive to – but not prejudiced against – the age, living circumstances, geographic location, disabilities, gender, culture, faith, personal relationships and lifestyle choices of service users. Care planning should build on the strengths and abilities of individuals and the part they can play in addressing their needs. It should address external or environmental factors that have caused the need to arise, or will hamper the resolutions of need if not addressed.
>
> (Department of Health, 2002e: 24)

Partnership working is therefore seen as beneficial and desirable as it can:

- improve the effectiveness of the care and support process;
- see service users and carers as a source of knowledge and understanding, which is fundamental to person-centred and individualised care;
- ensure that service user and carer rights remain central to the decision-making process;
- facilitate the process of empowerment for service users and carers.

(Hatton, 2008)

Partnership working and collaborative working differ, in that a 'partnership is a shared commitment to a course of action, where all partners have a right and an obligation to participate and will be affected equally by the benefits and disadvantages arising from the partnership' (Buchanan and Carnwell, 2005: 6), while collaborative working involves working jointly with each other, reflecting concepts of empowerment and anti-oppressive practice (Buchanan and Carnwell, 2005). Partnerships therefore can be about contractual arrangements, while collaboration is about the nature of the partnership and implies a shared agenda, vision and goals.

Ingredients for successful partnership with both other professionals and service users include:

- trust and respect;
- shared expertise (it is important to remember that the service user is expert in their lived experience);
- leadership;
- participation – non-hierarchical;
- shared responsibility and willingness to work together;
- strategies to overcome barriers;
- communication.

What kind of partnerships?

As stated above, partnerships exist between health, social care and service users and carers, reflecting a consumerist and empowering approach to care management. In addition, partnerships exist between health and social care agencies through joint agreements about the planning and delivery of services, as well as joint commissioning processes. The driver for this was seen in New Labour's health and social care policy on improving collaboration and was most evident in the formation of new integrated organisations called Care Trusts as proposed in the *NHS Plan* (DH, 2000a) and made mandatory in the Heath and Social

Care Act of 2001. The objective of Care Trusts was essentially to break down organisational boundaries and, importantly, to provide funding streams. The Care Trusts would then, in theory, become multi-purpose legal bodies that can commission and deliver health and social services for vulnerable groups leading to better collaboration and integration of those services (Crinson, 2008). However, such a single system approach has not been adopted wholesale with only 11 such Trusts in existence in England by the end of 2008, with NHS Trusts more likely to make specific endeavours in small jointly commissioned projects such as day care services.

Partnerships also exist in relation to local consultation exercises, where Local Authorities or the government seek to find out the views of service users and carers in line with the policy agenda to improve service user and carer involvement in decision-making processes at every level of care planning and delivery (see Chapter 2). This may be in relation to a specific issue or service, at either a micro or macro level. For example, at a micro level, the residents of a care home may be consulted about a change in the social events programme within the home, while at a macro level people may be consulted about a particular area of need. An example of this might be a specialist service, such as residential drug and alcohol treatment services, within a particular locality.

Types of partnership

Partnership and collaborative working is not particularly new to health and social care, but has been widely promoted as a desirable way to work to address needs and solve problems. Whittington (2003) identifies three broad ways in which working in partnership might operate.

1. Agencies working together to provide joined-up services.
2. Meeting service user needs through the provision of services by more than one organisation (for example, crossing the boundaries between health and social care agencies, statutory and independent care providers and voluntary organisations).
3. A collaborative relationship between care provider and the service user and carer.

Within the consumerist model of health care, with a focus on person-centred care and collaborative working, the concept of co-production is important. This reflects a power shift where service users are seen as active contributors to every stage of the ASPIRE process. The key elements of co-production are as follows:

- it emphasises that people are not passive recipients of services and have assets and expertise, which can help improve services;
- it is a potentially transformative way of thinking about power, resources, partnerships, risks and outcomes, not an off-the-shelf model of service provision or a single magic solution;
- it focuses on empowerment of both users and providers to act as partners in the care process – co-production means involving citizens in collaborative relationships with more empowered frontline staff who are able and confident to share power and accept user expertise;
- staff should be trained in the benefits of co-production, supported in positive risk taking and encouraged to identify new opportunities for collaboration with people who use services;
- people should be encouraged to access co-productive initiatives, recognising and supporting diversity among the people who use services;
- the creation of new structures, regulatory and commissioning practices and financial streams is necessary to embed co-production as a long-term rather than ad hoc solution;
- learning from existing international case studies of co-production while recognising the contribution of initiatives reflecting local needs is important.

(SCIE, 2008)

The nature of partnerships

Partnerships may be problem-orientated, ideological or ethical in nature. Problem-orientated partnerships address specific problems, which can be individual or service-related. An example of this type of partnership may be where a practitioner works with a service user to address a particular need and to achieve specific outcomes. Ideological partnerships are those partnerships where different individuals or agencies have a shared vision, agenda and goal, such as a reduction in the number of incidences of domestic violence, or the promotion of positive images of ageing (The Better Government for Older People Project was a partnership between statutory bodies, voluntary agencies, independent organisations and individuals who came together to devise a strategy to improve the experiences of ageing, see **www.bettergovernmentforolderpeople.org.uk**).

Ethical partnerships promote a particular perspective, which is of benefit to a wider population, such as the five-a-day campaign to promote increased consumption of fruit and vegetables for healthier eating and longer-term health benefits.

Level of involvement	Methods	Tasks
Informed.	Newsletters, leaflets, posters, radio.	Informing service users about entitlements, resources, new services.
Consultation.	Focus or discussion groups, semi-structured interviews, questionnaires.	Finding out views on services.
Collaboration/ partnership.	Committees, working groups.	Agreeing priorities for service improvements.
User control.	Self help and support groups, user groups.	Users decide priorities and action in response to need.

Table 19 Levels and methods of service user involvement (Oliviere, Hargreaves and Monroe, 1998)

Barriers to working in partnership

Activity

Think about a group or team that you have worked in.

1. What difficulties did you encounter in working together?
2. How might group work be sabotaged (either intentionally or unintentionally)?

While there are examples of good partnership working throughout the health and social care sector, there are also a number of barriers to effective partnership working. As argued in Chapter 2, increasing user and carer involvement in health and social care is a fundamental policy imperative. However, there are a number of different ways that users and carers can be involved in the decision-making processes in health and social care, involving different levels of partnership and empowerment. There are variations in the nature of collaborative working between different geographical localities and different service user and carer groups, and user and carer involvement in decision-making may be seen as tokenistic. Arnstein's ladder of empowerment (see Figure 13) is useful to illustrate this, identifying different ways of engaging users and carers and the degree to which this involves and empowers them (Arnstein, 1969).

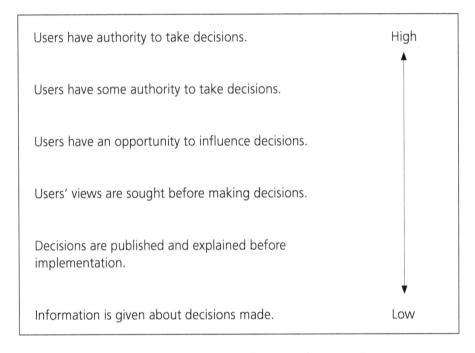

Figure 13 Levels of empowerment (Braye and Preston-Shoot, 1995)

For practitioners in health and social care, there may be a fear of loss of professional identity when working collaboratively with other health and social care practitioners as well as with service users and carers (Hudson, 2002). This may be particularly acute when working within the multi-disciplinary team, and sociological exploration of professions and power can help to explain this.

Professionalism

> ## Activity
>
> Examine the following characteristics of a profession:
>
> - the creation and defence of a specialist body of knowledge, typically based on formal university qualifications;
> - the establishment of control over a specialised client market and exclusion of competitor groups from that market;
> - the establishment of control over professional work practice, responsibilities and obligations while resisting control from managerial or bureaucratic staff.
>
> (Bilton *et al.*, 2002: 426)
>
> 1. How far could social work or nursing be argued to be a professional group based on the above criteria?

There are many theories of professionalism (Johnson, 1972), but a common way to describe a group as a profession is based on the acquisition of a number of characteristics or traits.

It can be argued that professionalism based on expert knowledge is concerned with power and control within an occupational hierarchy. Within the multi-disciplinary team there are inequalities in status and power within the different occupational groups (Lymbery, 2005), and this concept of relative power can impact on the nature of collaborative working. However, Dhalley (1989) provides a more positive assessment of collaborative working in teams, where beneficial alliances can be established through inter-disciplinary working, and Lymbery and Millward (2000) conclude that research demonstrates considerable improvements in inter-professional working.

There may also be barriers to effective partnership working where there is a lack of integration between different management and organisational structures. Incompatibility of goals may lead to difficulties in partnership working, and this may be compounded by the location of different practitioners. In their evaluation of an enablement project, Llewellyn and Mercer (2008) concluded that inter-professional collaboration was more successful when different occupational groups were located within the same geographical locality, facilitating improved communication and shared goal setting. However, different theoretical perspectives underpinning professional practice may lead to difficulties in collaborative working, as this leads to difficulties in establishing a collective vision and agenda and setting goals. For example, a professional culture that is risk averse may lead to difficulties in having a shared vision and objectives with a professional culture that promotes positive risk taking and enablement of individuals (Titterton, 2005).

Collaborative and partnership working also depend on good strategic leadership and positive role models throughout the hierarchical structures of the organisation. This is acknowledged in the government document *Putting People First* (DH, 2007b).

> The local authority and Director of Adult Social Services (DASS) have key strategic and leadership roles and work with a range of partners, including Primary Care Trusts (PCTs) and the independent and voluntary sectors, to provide services which are well planned and integrated, make the most effective use of available resources, and meet the needs of a diverse community.

In 2004, the Commission for Social Care Inspection found a number of barriers to partnership working in relation to the personalisation agenda that originated from Local Councils. These included a lack of information for service users and low staff awareness of new models of working and what they were trying to achieve. In addition, staff failed to empower some individuals because of their assumptions that they did not have the capacity or ability to manage their own budget. Processes of record keeping, which involved unnecessary and overly bureaucratic paperwork, were also seen as barriers to effective collaborative care. This demonstrates that everybody has a responsibility to work towards more effective collaborative working.

Smale *et al.* (1993) promote the exchange model of working as an effective way of working in partnership with service users and carers. Within this model, it is assumed that people:

- are experts in themselves.

In relation to practitioners it assumes that they:

- have expertise in the process of problem-solving with others;

- understand and share perceptions of problems with their management;
- will get agreement about who will do what to support whom;
- will take responsibility for arriving at the optimum resolution of problems within the constraints of available resources and the willingness of participants to contribute.

(Smale *et al.*, 1993: 18)

Effective collaborative and partnership working also depends on good record keeping and addressing issues of confidentiality.

WRITING CARE PLANS AND KEEPING RECORDS

Client records

Dimond (2005) states that, in principle, anything that relates to a client within the context of their care can be seen as part of their health care records. According to the Nursing and Midwifery Council (2009) record keeping has many important functions and these include a range of clinical, administrative and educational uses. These principles and functions should be related to social care records as well. Good records should:

- help to improve accountability;
- show how decisions related to patient care were made;
- support the delivery of services;
- support effective clinical judgements and decisions;
- support service user care and communications;
- make continuity of care easier;
- provide documentary evidence of services delivered;
- promote better communication and sharing of information between members of the multi-professional health care team;
- help to identify risks, enabling early detection of complications;
- support clinical audit, research, allocation of resources and performance planning;
- help to address complaints or legal processes.

Activity

The principles of good record keeping apply to all types of records, regardless of how they are held.

1. List 10 types of 'records' that may relate to a single client's care.

(Hint – It might be helpful to look at the guidance for nurses and midwives in the NMC website or the Data Protection Act 1998 or the Scottish Social Services Council guidance for social work students at **www4.rgu.ac.uk/files/Data%20Protection%20Notice%20 for%20Students_revised%20Apr08_.pdf**)

Employers usually set the way in which health and social care workers keep records and so different methods for planning care and keeping records are used. However, it is essential that the principles of good record keeping are used and that these reflect the core values of individuality and partnership working.

The Audit Commission make recommendations (see **www.audit-commission.gov.uk**) and the NMC has published guidance (2009) considering important issues such as:

- ensuring that records are signed and dated;
- writing records contemporaneously ensuring the accuracy and consistency of the record;
- ensuring that records are written clearly and in such a manner that they cannot be erased, with alterations dated, timed and signed so the author can be identified;
- not using jargon or abbreviations;
- not using subjective statements that could be offensive or speculative.

One other consideration is that if an episode of care is not recorded then there is no evidence that the care giving happened. The law would therefore tend to adopt the approach that if an assessment, interaction or intervention is not recorded it is not considered to have taken place

(Rogers, 2009). This might have implications for a practitioner who has to attend court and who may not be able to prove that they had complied with their duty to care.

Case study

While providing personal care to an elderly lady with dementia Bernadette, a care worker, notices that the lady has developed a small red patch on her left heel. She is convinced that it was not there when she last visited the lady three days ago. There is nothing noted in the care plan. Bernadette writes the following entry in the care plan:

Small red patch noted on left heel.

- How could this episode of record keeping be improved?
- What might you have recorded here?

Confidentiality, data and sharing information

One of the issues practitioners need to consider and address at all stages of ASPIRE, but particularly during the record keeping and planning stages, is the issue of confidentiality. Confidentiality is one of the most important rules of health care ethics as confidentiality of information demonstrates respect for the individual (Tschudin, 2006). In health and social care it is about protecting all information about the individual, and complying with the Human Rights Act (1998) as it relates to the right to privacy. Both the GSCC and the NMC require practitioners to maintain confidentiality of clients with disclosure only being justified if information is required by law.

Activity

Review either the NMC *Code* or the GSCC *Code of Practice for Social Workers* and see what they state about your professional duty to protect confidentiality.

Confidentiality is particularly pertinent when considering the sharing of records through the Single Assessment Process and Common Assessment Framework as it further develops. The sharing of information across health and social care supports multi-disciplinary assessment and planning, and can lead to individuals getting the support that underpins their independence and achieving the outcomes they want for their lives by enabling choice. If information collected at different sources can be drawn together it can save time and also address practical issues such as individuals needing to repeat information to a number of different professionals. The proliferation of IT over the last two decades has therefore brought new opportunities and new challenges to keeping records.

Practitioners need to be fully aware of the legal requirements and guidance regarding confidentiality and ensure practice is in line with national and local policies when keeping and storing records. Consideration should be given to any information that can identify a person in your care as it must not be used or disclosed for purposes other than health and social care without the individual's explicit consent. The exception to this is that you can release this information if the law requires it, or where there is a wider public interest.

There are a number of central elements that need to be taken into consideration that underpin information sharing and these are listed within the Department of Health's Consultation Document *Common Assessment Framework for Adults* (DH, 2009d).

- The individual's **consent** to having their personal details shared needs to be explicit in terms of what the information is and with whom it should and should not be shared.
- Any sharing of an individual's personal information needs to be on the basis that it is **secure** and can only be accessed, with appropriate consent, by professionals who have a legitimate interest in that person's support.
- The mechanism should allow secure patient and user access, and potentially direct control of the information.
- Information sharing should support an individual approach and be clearly set within the context of the personal outcomes that a person wants in their own life.
- There should be a link to and from wider specialist assessments, as well as any other assessments such as web-based self-assessments for equipment.

- It should allow people to frame their own overall assessment and care planning needs, by themselves, with their carers and/or with professional support and advice.
- It should allow the sharing of a limited amount of information that is up-to-date and correct, in a way that is helpful and useful to the different professionals who may be involved.
- There should perhaps be different views of the information, detail and background, since different professional groups (such as GPs, community nurses or physiotherapists) are likely to want to see a different initial view or cut of information held.
- The mechanism should provide the basis for recording the information once.

Thus, while the opportunity of a national IT network, with the possibility of sharing records between professionals and across professions and services, is valuable, it is important to make consideration of the security of IT systems. The security measures such as smartcards or passwords to access information systems must not be shared, or systems left open to access when you have finished using them, or unauthorised individuals will be able to access confidential information.

However, computer-held records do offer a number of advantages in addition to information sharing. These include the ability to audit care and to use templates and standardised planning to improve the approach to care planning and record keeping. Using data to audit records does however highlight the importance of data quality. The quality of information from systems is only as good as the information that goes into a system. Shared standards, common coding and an agreement across professional groups not to replicate data are crucial to its success.

It is also important to remember that people in our care have the legal right to ask to see their own health records. Different public sector organisations will have local policies, which you must be aware of, and organisations employing health and social care staff will have policy and guidelines to address this right.

Activity

1. Find your local policy on health and social care record keeping and sharing.
2. List the key principles of the policy.

Equally, it is important that people in your care are told that information on their records may be seen by other people or agencies involved in their care but, also, that they have the right to ask for their information to be withheld from you or other professionals. This should be discussed as part of the assessment process and consent gained or otherwise. Requests to withhold information must be respected unless withholding such information would cause serious harm to that person or others as, under common law, you are allowed to disclose information if it will help to prevent, detect, investigate or punish serious crime or if it will prevent abuse or serious harm to others.

It is important that, as well as considering issues of securing records, practitioners make sure that confidentiality is also applied to all areas of practice. For example, it is essential that discussions concerning the people in your care are not conducted in places where you might be overheard. This applies to areas in your place of work just as it does when outside work like, for example, on the bus on the way home. It is equally important that records, either on paper or on computer screens, are not left or placed where they might be seen by unauthorised staff or members of the public. Finally, you should not access the records of any person, or their family, to find out personal information that is not relevant to their care.

THE PRACTICALITIES OF CARE PLANNING

It must be acknowledged at this stage that care planning can be very complex. Planning relies on the interpersonal skills of the professional working with the client in order to fully hear what their wants and needs are, and working within the therapeutic relationship to ensure partnership is achieved (see Chapter 6). There is, however, another consideration to be made and that is about the issue of resources.

The funding of health and social care services is a huge political pressure, with a significant portion of Gross Domestic Product (the total value of all goods and products made within a year as a measure of a country's economic performance) being committed to running the NHS (£118 billion on health care in 2007, 8.4 per cent of GDP (Office for National Statistics, 2009). The seemingly exponential rise of the cost of medical technologies, a year on year increase in the number of prescriptions (DH, 2002c), and the increasing use of novel medical technological improvements that are often more expensive than the procedures they replace (Bradshaw and Bradshaw, 2004), are a source of financial pressure for the NHS. The government attempts, through the arms-length body the

National Institute of Health and Clinical Excellence (NICE), to control the use of medicines and technological advances through the publication of guidelines (see Chapter 7), but these costs continue to rise.

Similarly, social care provision operates within a context of scarce resources and delivery of public sector services is based on eligibility criteria. Within a marketised system of welfare provision, there is a tension for the social work and social care role between the provision of person-centred care based on needs-led assessment and the planning and management of scarce resources (Wilson *et al.*, 2008).

It is thus an imperative part of the planning stage of ASPIRE to plan care based on local and national guidance. This should be based on current evidence and consideration of the financial envelope open to the services in question. Evidence-based interventions will be discussed in more detail in Chapter 6.

Activity

Think back to the case study about Stuart on page 139. Referring to national guidance on the treatment of obesity and carrying out research using the internet, identify the estimated cost of obesity to the UK in terms of morbidity and associated medical and social effects, for example lost working days. Considering these costs do you think that addressing obesity should be a priority for services? Are there any evidence-based (and therefore cost-effective) treatments or interventions for obesity?

SUMMARY

Building on the assessment chapter, Chapter 5 has examined the nature of planning care and support, looking at both goal setting and the use of SMART objectives and MACROS, and why this is important within a phased approach to planning the care process. Partnership working within the multi-disciplinary team and through collaborative working with service users and carers has been explored within the context of a resource-constrained service. The importance of keeping accurate written records and confidentiality has been discussed. The role of information technology in health and social care has been considered, as well as the implications of the increased use of IT within health and social care.

Reflection	
Identify at least three things that you have learned from this chapter.	1. 2. 3.
How do you plan to use this knowledge in care practice?	1. 2. 3.
How will you evaluate the effectiveness of your plan?	1. 2. 3.
What further knowledge and evidence do you need?	1. 2. 3.

FURTHER READING

Leathard, A. and McLaren, S. (Ed) (2007) *Ethics: Contemporary Challenges in Health and Social Care.* Cambridge: Polity Press

This book examines theory, research, policy and practice in both health and social care fields. The importance of this approach is reflected in the growing emphasis on ethical issues in research and practice and, in Britain, on government policy aimed at improving partnership working across the two sectors. The analysis is set within the context of contemporary challenges facing health and social care, not only in Britain but internationally. Contributors from the UK, US and Australia consider: ethical issues in health and social care research and governance; inter-professional and user perspectives; ethics in relation to human rights, the law, finance, management and provision; key issues of relevance to vulnerable groups, such as children and young people, those with complex disabilities, older people and those with mental health problems; and life-course issues – ethical perspectives on a range of challenging areas from new technologies of reproduction to euthanasia.

Marquis, B. and Huston, C. (2008) *Leadership Roles and Management Functions in Nursing: Theory and Application.* London: Lippincott

Now in its Sixth Edition, this key leadership and management text incorporates application with theory and emphasises critical thinking, problem-solving and decision-making. More than 225 case studies and learning exercises promote critical thinking and interactive discussion. Case studies cover a variety of settings, including acute care, ambulatory care, long-term care, and community health. The book addresses timely issues such as leadership development, staffing, delegation, ethics and law, organisational, political, and personal power, management and technology, and more. Web links and learning exercises appear in each chapter.

Chapter 6

Intervention

This chapter covers the following key issues:

- the nature of intervention in health and social care;
- types of health and social care intervention;
- evidence-based interventions;
- working in partnership to enable intervention activity;
- advocacy.

By the end of this chapter you should be able to:

- articulate the reasons and rationale for undertaking different types of interventions in health and social care;
- discuss the importance of working in partnership to implement care;
- identify the importance of culturally appropriate caring;
- reflect on what role health and social care practitioners have in advocacy.

This chapter matches to the following National Occupational Standards and Essential Skills Clusters:

- ESC 2.iii Actively encourages patient/client to be involved in, and/or ensures they are supported in own care/self-care;
- ESC 2.vi Provides care (or makes provisions) for those who are unable to maintain own personal care;
- ESC 3.iv Delivers care with dignity, making appropriate use of the environment, self, skills and attitudes;
- ESC 3.vi Acts in a way that demonstrates respect for others, promoting and valuing differences;
- ESC 4.iii Adopts a principled approach to care underpinned by the NMC code;
- ESC 5 Provide care that is delivered in a warm, sensitive and compassionate way;

- ESC 10 Deliver and evaluate care against the comprehensive assessment and care plan;
- ESC 18 Identify and safely manage risk in relation to the patient/ client, the environment, self and others.
- NOS 5.3 Apply and justify social work methods and models used to achieve change and development, and improve life opportunities;
- NOS 6.3 Carry out your own responsibilities and monitor, co-ordinate and support the actions of others involved in implementing the plans;
- NOS 10.3 Advocate for and with individuals, families, carers, groups and communities;
- NOS 14.2 Carry out duties using accountable professional judgement and knowledge-based social work practice.

INTRODUCTION

The intervention phase of the care process is concerned with the provision of care and the implementation of the care plan. There are three key issues that need to be considered when discussing intervention:

1. how the care will be implemented;
2. the nature of the intervention;
3. who provides care.

Person-centred care

We live in a diverse society, with a plurality of beliefs among individuals, families and members of social groups. Person-centred care is practice that recognises the circumstances, concerns, goals, beliefs and cultures of the individual, their family and friends. Each individual is unique and has unique needs, so it is important to acknowledge the significance of spiritual, emotional and religious support.

> Care is delivered in a sensitive, person-centred way that takes account of the circumstances, wishes and priorities of the individual, their family and friends.
>
> National End of Life Care Strategy available at **www. endoflifecareforadults.nhs.uk/eolc** (last accessed 23.10.09)

There are a number of different ways and processes of delivering care that can make a difference to a person's life and address their needs. Within a holistic framework of care, interventions can focus on making a difference in the physical, psychological, social, spiritual and/or environmental domains of a person's life. Maslow's (1954) hierarchy of needs (see Figure 14) is a useful framework to demonstrate the levels of need that care interventions might focus on to improve a care recipient's health and social wellbeing.

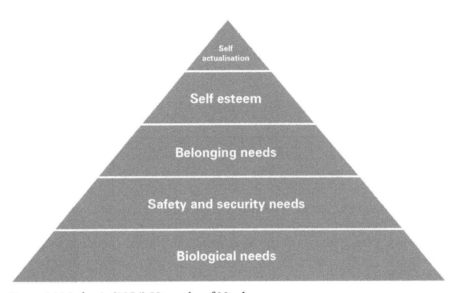

Figure 14 Maslow's (1954) Hierarchy of Needs

Activity

Refer back to the case study about Frank on pages 19-20. Can you identify his needs using Maslow's Hierarchy of Needs?

Biological needs are fundamental to a person's wellbeing and capacity to achieve their maximum potential within a holistic concept of self (see Chapter 1). Interventions to address biological needs are sometimes referred to as basic care (Henderson, 1960). However, this can be misleading as the term 'basic' can be misconstrued as menial. The provision of good quality and timely interventions to address biological needs is a highly skilled activity, involving the use of a range of psychomotor and interpersonal skills to provide care in an individualised manner that respects the care recipient's dignity and self-worth.

INTERVENTIONS

Interventions may be designed to focus primarily on a specific task, although assessment of need should have been conducted within a holistic framework. Thus, interventions may be based on the planned achievement of certain goals, or they may be implemented to address a specific crisis.

Task-centred interventions

In nursing practice, up until 1972, at least 61 per cent of nursing interventions in the acute hospital setting were based on the allocation of tasks (Pearson, 1988). Task allocation involved the breaking down of care into specific tasks, such as bathing, feeding or provision of medications, and these would be allocated to individual nurses. So, for example, one nurse would do all the washing and bathing, while another would dispense all medications. Once the task had been completed, the nurse would withdraw from the patient and move on to the next task. This system of intervention has its roots in the development of nursing within the army and church, where the emphasis was on authority and the hierarchical division of tasks. It was seen as efficient and cost-effective (Pearson, 1988) and continued to be widely used long after nursing became a secular occupation. Hayward (1975) found that nurses would feel guilty if they stayed and talked to a patient after the task had been completed, while Menzies (1960) takes this a step further, arguing that this system of task allocation prevented nurses from becoming too involved with the patient and helped them to retain a social distance and protect themselves from emotional engagement.

Task allocation as a system of intervention in nursing practice has been widely criticised as it leads to a fragmentation of care and a lack of focus on the holistic care of the individual. It could also be argued that it is less satisfying for the practitioner, who engages in a series of repetitive tasks rather than utilising a range of skills and knowledge to achieve holistic care. As stated previously, the provision of care is an interpersonal activity, and the focus on the division of labour and the allocation of tasks militates against person-centred and individualised care, reducing the care task to an assembly line type activity, with a focus on outcome at the expense of quality and process.

Activity

Xavier, aged 35, has just returned to the ward following abdominal surgery to remove a malignant growth in his large intestine. He is to remain nil by mouth and has an intravenous drip. He requires frequent observation of his vital signs and wound, and he has a temporary colostomy.

1. List the tasks of care intervention that Xavier will require.
2. Consider how you would feel if you were the care recipient here and had a range of different practitioners performing these various tasks of care.

Although this method of organising interventions has been criticised, task-centred approaches can be an effective method of health and social care intervention (Parker and Bradley, 2003), which provide an effective and practical method of intervention with service users. The emphasis is on setting short, achievable goals in partnership with service users so that desired changes can be achieved, although task-centred approaches can also be used when service users are reluctant to work collaboratively or do not have the capacity to negotiate decisions and goals (for example, when the patient is unconscious).

The task-centred approach to social work practice draws on theoretical perspectives of problem-solving and behavioural approaches, and can be seen to be very similar to cognitive and behavioural approaches that are used within mental health practice (Lindsay, 2009; Fawcett and Karban, 2005). Reid and Epstein (1972) identify the following areas of social work practice where a task-centred approach would be useful:

- interpersonal conflict;
- dissatisfaction in social relations;
- relations with formal organisations;
- role performance;
- social transition;
- reactive emotional distress;
- inadequate resources.

Crisis intervention

Crisis intervention approaches are also often used in health and social care work. They have their roots in developmental psychology and cognitive behavioural psychology but, in reality, draw on a range of different theoretical perspectives (McGinnis, 2009). Often, when people engage with health and social care services, they are experiencing some sort of crisis (whether it is interpersonal, physical, emotional, spiritual or social or a combination). Stress is an important concept to consider here – the ways in which we help people to manage the stressors that they are experiencing and work with their own resilience and coping strategies. We all experience stress throughout our lives and find ways to manage this stress. It is when the stress is unmanageable, either because of the unusual nature of it (as in physical crisis) or because of the severity, duration or a multiplicity of stressors, that a person may require intervention from health and social care practitioners.

Activity

Think about a recent stressful event that you experienced (this might be something like a new social encounter or engaging with a new and unfamiliar task).

1. How did the stress make you feel?
2. How did you manage the stress and cope with the situation?
3. What skills did you draw on from your experience of coping in previous stressful encounters?

Crisis interventions operate within systems theory, where the care recipient is seen as a system of inter-related parts within a wider social and environmental system (see the section on systems models of nursing in Chapter 5). Various methods of intervention can be used to manage the crisis, including psychosocial and cognitive behavioural, psychotherapeutic, family therapy, problem-solving approaches and solution-focused approaches, depending on the nature of the crisis and the desired outcome. It is beyond the scope of this book to discuss these approaches in detail (see Lindsay, 2009 for a more detailed discussion).

Safeguarding vulnerable individuals is an important aspect of crisis intervention. This might sometimes involve invoking safeguarding procedures in order to ensure that they are protected from abusive or neglectful environments. Procedures and policies for intervention where there is suspected or alleged abuse or neglect are set out in statute in The Children Act for children and in the *No Secrets* guidance for vulnerable adults (DH, 2002b) (see Chapter 3).

Diagnostic interventions

Diagnostic interventions are those interventions that help to determine a course of action or help to maintain the safety of the service user. There is some overlap here with the assessment phase of the care process, although diagnostic interventions will also form a distinct part of the process. Lindberg *et al.* (1990) identify the following key elements of diagnostic intervention.

1. **Observation** – practitioners are constantly observing the people they work with for changes in their condition, including observation of vital signs, appearance, non-verbal communications, such as signs of pain or anxiety, responses to medication and any observable side effects. In addition, practitioners will observe service users for signs of risk and the need for protection and safeguarding. Some high profile cases have emphasised the need for good observation when safeguarding vulnerable people, such as the death of Baby Peter (*Laming Report*, DH, 2009e), as professionals involved in his care were criticised for failing to observe or interpret signs of abuse and neglect.

2. **Inspection** – there is a clear role for practitioners to examine service users for any changes in their condition. This could include, for example, the inspection of a wound or pressure sore to detect any improvements or deteriorations (see also Chapter 7 regarding evaluation). In addition, professionals are also involved in inspection to ensure that vulnerable people are safeguarded from abuse and neglect.

   > There is a clear need for a determined focus on improvement of practice in child protection across all the agencies that support children. New ways should be created to share good practice and learn lessons when things go wrong. Within that context there is a need to strengthen the inspection processes of each of the services responsible for the safety of children. Inspection should not be a stand-alone activity. It should not be only an isolated snapshot. It must be accompanied by a robust developmental process aimed at achieving higher standards of service provision.
   >
   > (*Laming Report*, 2009e: 61)

3. **Monitoring** – this involves checking on a regular basis and is an effective intervention in preventative practice. For example, dentists monitor the condition of teeth through regular check-ups, while health visitors and school nurses monitor child growth and development. Individuals may also self-monitor, for example a person with diabetes may monitor their blood glucose level or urinary glucose on a regular basis, while someone on a reducing diet may weigh themselves on a weekly basis. Self monitoring and self evaluation are fundamental to changes in health care practice, which emphasise person-centred care and the notion of the service user as the expert in their own care as identified within the Department of Health's *Expert Patient Programme* (DH, 2008c).

The *Expert Patient Programme* was launched in 2008 following a successful pilot in 2002 and it is designed to help people with long-term conditions manage their own condition. This not only empowers them and fosters a greater degree of independence, but also leads to a better quality of life. The aims of the *Expert Patient Programme* are that service users should:

- feel confident and in control of their lives;
- aim to manage their condition and its treatment in partnership with health care professionals;
- communicate effectively with professionals and be willing to share responsibility on treatment;
- be realistic about the impact of their disease on themselves and their family, and
- use their skills and knowledge to lead full lives.

(DH, 2008c)

4. **Listening** – a number of diagnostic tools can be used to listen for signs and changes in conditions, such as stethoscopes, doplar and sonicaid (for example, stethoscopes may be used for listening to an individual's chest for signs of chest infection; doplar tools use a form of ultrasound pulsing to listen for signs such as pedal pulses; sonicaid is another tool for listening and is often used in antenatal care to listen for the baby's heart beat while in the uterus). The practitioner's own listening skills are also important and can be used to listen for non-verbalised signs. For example, a practitioner may be able to pick up on anxiety, pain and suffering through listening to the changes in voice, and practitioners are increasingly encouraged through models of professional practice to listen to what the service users and carers have to say.

Therapeutic interventions

Therapeutic interventions are those interventions that maintain the strengths and coping abilities of the service user and carer, as well as treating problems. Therapeutic interventions involve a range of helping skills and can be used for a variety of reasons, such as meeting basic needs, helping people to develop their own skills, assisting with activities of daily living and problem-solving. Therapeutic interventions can also be used to demonstrate caring and to provide relaxation and improve self-esteem. For example, Tutton (1991) identifies touch as a way of communicating care and wellbeing. In this sense, touch can convey messages of acceptance and trust and can therefore be therapeutic. In addition, Routasalo (1998) concludes that touch can be therapeutic when it has a calming and comforting effect on a service user.

Health education and health promotion are also important therapeutic interventions and reflect the contemporary policy agenda in relation to prevention of disease and illness (see Chapter 2). Public health initiatives, which consist of delivering health promotion programmes, can be key interventions in enabling the prevention of disease, disability or illness and health and social care practitioners are in a key position to deliver this type of intervention (Coverdale, 2009). Health promotion is, on the one hand, the prevention and control of premature death and disease and, on the other, the promotion of wellbeing and control over health. This can be achieved through both empowering and enabling individuals, which helps to make healthy choices easier (Tones and Green, 2004). Intervention can take place at an individual level where service users are enabled to understand their disease or disability better through access to information, education or services, or when they are enabled to explore the ways in which they can cope with their circumstances by one-to-one intervention with a single practitioner. Intervention can also take place at population level. This may include a host of health-promoting campaigns such as the child immunisation programme or media campaigns delivering health messages such as the Fit4life campaign, and may involve building health promotion activities into a care plan for an individual like, for example, 'quit smoking' interventions or interventions to promote safe sexual activity.

Activity

Think back over the previous 10–15 years of your life. Can you think of any health education or health-promoting activities that you yourself will have been influenced by (for example, at school or at home)?

Case study

Michelle is a 25-year-old woman with learning disabilities who lives with her parents. You have been providing support to Michelle and her family for some time. Her mother rings you to tell you that Michelle has started a sexual relationship and 'it has to stop'. She is concerned that Michelle is being 'taken advantage of' and that her boyfriend is abusive towards her. She says that her daughter should not be allowed to have a sexual relationship.

To find out more information, you speak to a worker at the day centre that Michelle attends. The worker informs you that they are aware of the sexual relationship she is having. However, they do not feel comfortable speaking to Michelle about this and don't think this is something that they should deal with. The worker is not clear if Michelle is being abused in any way.

You arrange to see Michelle. Michelle becomes distressed when you broach the subject of her new relationship. She does not seem clear about sexual protection issues. You notice that she has a large bruise on her arm. When you ask Michelle about this she says she tripped over on the stairs.

1. How would you assess Michelle's needs and what types of interventions would your plan include?

Issues that you might consider:

- investigative skills to assess whether abuse is taking place;
- interventions to safeguard Michelle if abuse is taking place;
- interventions to assess capacity;
- information about alternative decisions;

- health education/health promotion about safe sex for Michelle (relating to unwanted pregnancy/sexually transmitted diseases);
- support for Michelle to make decisions if she has capacity;
- support for Michelle's parents;
- education and training for day centre staff;
- communication skills to develop a relationship of trust with Michelle and her parents;
- health education/health promotion about safe sex and consensual sex for Michelle's boyfriend.

Interventions therefore can be performed in a variety of ways, depending on the intended outcome. Contemporary policy imperatives stress the importance of early intervention and interventions aimed at preventing problems occurring (DH, 2009f). This can be seen within the wider policy context as discussed in Chapters 2 and 3. Tanner and Harris (2008) demonstrate this in relation to older people, where they identify the range of interventions that can promote wellbeing and independent living (see Figure 15).

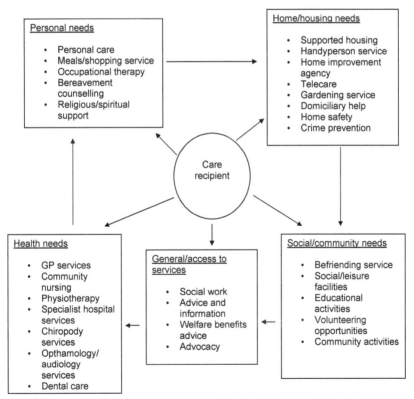

Figure 15 Examples of services to support wellbeing (Tanner and Harris, 2008: 94)

Effective interventions can take a number of forms and it is important that the appropriate intervention is used to address the needs as identified in the assessment process and to achieve the specific aims of the care plan. It is also important that interventions are based on a sound evidence base.

EVIDENCE-BASED PRACTICE

Interventions should be based on sound theoretical knowledge. They must be based on a proven (wherever possible) evidence base and, although evidence-based practice (EBP) appears at first glance to be more evident within health care, its principles apply equally to health and social care practices.

There is a plethora of definitions of evidence-based practice, from those that feel distinctly medical, to those involving professional judgement of some kind, and those recognising the implicit nature of involving the individual patient or care recipient (see Table 20). Also, there are definitions that recognise the importance of the effective use of resources and that EBP has to be actively pursued and managed.

Sackett *et al.*'s definition (1996) that EBP can be defined as 'the integration of best research evidence with expertise and patient (or client) values' incorporates three principles of practice that are required to optimise clinical (and non-clinical) outcomes but also, importantly, quality of life. The three principles are therefore:

1. relevant research;
2. the ability of the practitioner to use clinical (and non clinical) skills and past experiences to support each individual person's unique health state, their individual risks and benefits with regard to potential interventions and their personal values and expectations;
3. and the uniqueness, concerns and preferences that each patient brings which must be integrated into care decisions.

Sackett *et al.* (1996) argue that EBP comprises of five steps, which are:

1. converting the need for information into an answerable question;
2. tracking down the best evidence with which to answer that question;
3. critically appraising that evidence for its validity and applicability;
4. integrating the critical appraisal with our clinical expertise and with our patient's individuality;
5. evaluating the effectiveness and efficiency in executing steps 1–4 and seeking ways to improve them both next time (see Chapter 7).

Context or 'feel'	Definitions
EBP as distinctly medical.	Evidence-based medicine is the use of mathematical estimates of the risk of benefit and harm, derived from high quality research on population samples, to inform clinical decision-making in the diagnosis, investigation or management of individual service users. (Greenhalgh, 2000)
EBP as involving professional judgement of some kind.	The conscientious, explicit and judicious use of current-based evidence in making decisions about the care of individual service users. The practice of evidence-based medicine means integrating individual clinical expertise with the best available external clinical evidence from systematic research. (Sackett *et al.*, 1996)
EBP as recognising the implicit nature of involving the individual patient or care recipient involved.	Evidence-based clinical practice is an approach to decision-making in which the clinician uses the best evidence available, in consultation with the patient, to decide upon the option which suits that patient best. (Muir Gray, 1997)
Effective use of resources.	The process of systematically finding, appraising and using contemporaneous research findings as a basis for clinical decisions. It aims to eliminate the use of expensive, ineffective and dangerous medical decision-making. (Lockett, 1997)
Active pursuit and management of EBP.	Evidence-based practice has grown out of the desire by practitioners and managers that services that are provided are based on the best research evidence available. (Law, 2000)

Table 20 Definitions of evidence-based practice

It is important to acknowledge that evidence-based practice is the responsibility of all professionals, as colleagues of all skill mixes and experience can provide new evidence to influence practice. It is in the best interest of patients/clients to continuously question what we know and do and to change practices where there is an indication that they can be improved on. EBP is about:

- doing what works (does more good than harm);
- doing what is (or is most) effective;
- doing what works best (does most good);
- doing what is most cost-effective (does most good per £ spent);
- doing what is most efficient (timely);
- doing what raises patient/client 'satisfaction'.

However, it is also important to acknowledge that there is not an evidence base for all practice and this is where the concept of Best Practice fits in. Best Practice refers to practice where the technique, method, process, activity or, intervention is agreed to be the most efficient (least amount of effort) and effective (best results) way of accomplishing a task, based on the experience and agreement of expert practitioners.

SKILLS FOR INTERVENTION

Beresford (2007) identified the key elements that service users value in their relationships with professionals, and concluded that a social approach to intervention is seen as particularly beneficial, stressing the importance of the inter-relationship and the qualities of:

- warmth;
- respect;
- a non-judgemental approach;
- listening;
- treating people with equality;
- trustworthiness;
- an open and honest approach;
- reliability;
- good communication skills.

Service users value practitioners who give them time to sort things out for themselves and who provide support for them to work out their own agendas (Beresford, 2007), and thus diagnostic interventions are an important element of collaborative working and empowerment (see Chapter 5).

A person's mind and emotions are windows to the soul. Nursing care can be and is physical, procedural, objective, and factual, but at the highest level of nursing the nurses' human care responses, the human care transactions and the nurses' presence in the relationship transcend the physical and material world . . . and make contact with the person's emotional and subjective world as the route to the inner self . . .

(Watson, 1985: 50)

Dignity and respect

The right to be treated with dignity and respect is a fundamental human right and is enshrined in the Human Rights Act (1998). In November 2006, Ivan Lewis (MP), who was Minister for Care Services, launched the *Dignity in Care Campaign* in health and social care. The important principle being that:

> High quality health and social care services should be delivered in a person-centred way that respects the dignity of the individual receiving them.
>
> (DH, *Dignity in Care*, 2006c) **www.dh.gov.uk/en/SocialCare/ Socialcarereform/Dignityincare/index.htm**

One way of considering this is to give individual practitioners a framework within which to work such as the SCIE *Challenges for Dignity in Care* (2006).

- Zero tolerance for all forms of abuse.
- Support people with the same respect you would want for yourself or a member of your family.
- Treat each person as an individual by offering a personalised service.
- Enable people to maintain the maximum possible level of independence, choice and control.
- Listen and support people to express their needs and wants.
- Respect people's right to privacy.
- Ensure people feel able to complain without fear of retribution.
- Engage with family members and carers as care partners.
- Assist people to maintain confidence and a positive self-esteem.
- Act to alleviate people's loneliness and isolation.

Health and social care practitioners have privileged access to people's minds and bodies at a time when they may be feeling vulnerable.

Activity

Think about a practice encounter that you have had recently.

1. List the interventions that you engaged in.
2. In what ways did you have privileged access to the individual?

In 2007, the Health Care Commission identified a number of areas where care interventions did not treat older people with dignity:

- patients were addressed in an inappropriate manner or spoken about as if they were not there;
- people were not given information or did not have their consent sought or wishes considered;
- people were left in soiled clothes or exposed in an embarrassing manner;
- appropriate food or help with eating was not given;
- people were placed in mixed-sex accommodation.

It is therefore imperative that health and social care practitioners are aware of the impact of care on individuals and build up a relationship of trust so that interventions can be carried out in a sensitive and competent manner, according to the service user's wishes and best interests.

Culturally relevant and appropriate care

Care is organised around the needs and circumstances of the individual, and is delivered in a co-ordinated manner across services. It is delivered in a way that demonstrates respect for the individual, their family and friends, maintaining their dignity at all times. Workers are sensitive to circumstances, and their changing nature, and care is delivered accordingly.

National End of Life Care Strategy available at **www.endoflifecareforadults.nhs.uk/eolc** (last accessed 23.10.09)

The UK today is a 'multicultural, multiethnic and multiple language society' (Meddings and Haith-Cooper, 2008), and so the provision of culturally appropriate and relevant care interventions is a fundamental issue for health and social care professionals. Culture is made up of beliefs, values and ideas about what is right and what is wrong and these guide a person's behaviours or customs (Richardson, 2009). It is important that caregivers explore the ways in which they can provide appropriate care to individuals whose ethnic, cultural and race backgrounds are different to their own. Indeed, professional codes of conduct and organisational policies and guidelines will make it very clear to health and social care staff that ignorance of cultural needs or prejudicial attitudes are not acceptable.

Culture, ethnicity and race

Fernando (2001) argues that culture is characterised by a person's upbringing and choices, which lead to behaviours and attitudes that can be changed by, for example, adapting to different cultures. He characterises ethnicity as a sense of belonging and group identity determined by group pressures and psychological need. Race is characterised by physical appearance and genetic history, which can be argued to be as irrelevant as hair or eye colour (adapted from Richardson, 2009).

Activity

Think of your own ethnic/cultural background.

1. What differences of behaviour or attitudes can you list within your own ethnic or cultural 'group'? Think about religion, sexual orientation, diet, etc.
2. Think about your parents or grandparents. How is your behaviour culturally different from that of previous generations?

The attitude of a professional towards a care recipient, demonstrated through their professional caring behaviours, should display attributes of commitment, knowledge, skills and respect for the person, enabling the person to feel cared about (Stockdale and Warelow, 2000). Part of this as a process is about feeling accepted, i.e. worthy of dignity and respect, intrinsically valuable and precious as a human being (Brilowski and Wendler, 2005). Core to this caring relationship is Egan's concept of unconditional acceptance: that of accepting clients as individuals entitled to respect and care but not necessarily accepting their values and behaviours, which may be at odds with your own value systems (Egan, 2002).

This principle of unconditional acceptance enables culturally appropriate and relevant care giving, as cultural competency is important at both institutional and individual levels. Cross *et al.* (1989) identify five elements that are important in the provision of culturally competent care (see Table 21).

1. Valuing diversity.

2. Having the capacity for cultural self-assessment.

3. Being conscious of the dynamics inherent when cultures interact.

4. Having institutionalised cultural knowledge.

5. Having developed adaptations of service delivery reflecting an understanding of cultural diversity.

Table 21 Essential elements of culturally competent care (source: Cross, *et al.* 1989)

It is, however, also important for health and social care practitioners to acknowledge that it is not enough simply to understand the care recipient's culture – they must also have an awareness of the impact of their own cultural norms on their care giving by developing their knowledge of self through reflection. This will help the individual to recognise and address feelings about 'difference' that they may not even have recognised before, but which may have played a part in subconscious behaviours which challenge an individual's ability to achieve unconditional acceptance. If left unaddressed this can lead to discrimination (Richardson, 2009).

There are many situations within the care encounter where cultural differences impact and these could include:

- **personal space** – some cultures are comfortable with physical closeness, seeing it as a sign of caring, while others may prefer caregivers to maintain a physical distance whenever possible;
- **eye contact** – direct eye contact can be interpreted as aggressive or impolite and so, if an individual avoids eye contact, it may not mean that they are uninterested or shy but that they are demonstrating respect;
- **physical contact** – some cultures avoid contact with members of the opposite gender and may be very concerned with modesty and value being covered up even when being examined;

- **diet** – some cultures and religions prohibit certain foods and products containing food derivatives (for example, pork-derived insulin).

(Hayes and Llewellyn, 2008, p. 204)

Activity

Think about your own culture.

1. Describe your beliefs concerning personal space, eye contact, physical contact and diet.
2. How would you feel if someone challenged these beliefs?

While paying attention to cultural issues in care is important, it is also essential to acknowledge that, although identifying a care recipient as belonging to a cultural minority group may be useful as you are identifying their beliefs, values and customs, such an emphasis on group can also be problematic (Richardson, 2009). It is important to avoid creating stereotypes or assumptions about a person's culture, based on your perceptions of the group they belong to, rather than asking them about themselves and their needs. Individuality and valuing the individual remains the principle here.

Citizenship

The overarching principle of advocacy is that each person has a value, the capacity to grow and develop and (importantly) to participate. It fits within the context of 'society', which gives rise to human and legal rights and the concept of citizenship.

Citizenship is related to notions of freedom to participate within society, through the political and civil processes as well as through social and economic processes. Thus, the rights of citizenship are affected by inequalities in provision and quality of education, healthcare, housing, transport and other social amenities as well as inequalities in ability to participate in economic life. In addition citizenship is related to the ability to participate in the consumer market. Furthermore, the rights of citizenship are related to freedoms from victimisation and abuse (Bochel et al., 2005). Thus racial victimisation, domestic violence, elder abuse and child abuse can all limit people's freedoms. Justice is related to freedom and citizenship within a democratic society.

(Llewellyn et al., 2008)

Examining different forms of citizenship can help to uncover the rights that health and social care practitioners must consider in care situations.

Rights to:	Denial of citizenship
Freedom of speech and association.	Criminal victimisation.
Freedom from discrimination.	Racial harassment.
Protection of the law (for self and property).	Limited political participation.
	Erosion of legal right (to silence, to counsel, to fair trial, to trial by jury).
	Denial of protection under public order laws and civil liberties.

Table 22 Civil and political citizenship

Activity

Consider your professional group. How does your employer legislate to ensure the rights of your service users are protected?

Rights to:	Denial of citizenship
Education.	Inequalities in provision and quality of education, healthcare, housing, transport and social amenities.
Housing.	Unemployment.
Health care.	Underemployment and low pay.
Own property.	Erosion of benefit levels.
Consume goods and services.	Restricted access to welfare benefits.
Work and participation in economic life.	Policing of (and for) the family.
An income (welfare rights).	

Table 23 Social and economic citizenship

Activity

Consider how current government legislation has supported this aspect of citizenship – for example, the minimum wage, access to health care, etc.

Rights to:	Denial of citizenship
The benefits, in amenity and in health, of a safe and clean environment.	Poverty.
	Sickness and disease.
	Mortality.
	Geographies of despair.
	Urban and rural pollution.

Table 24 Environmental citizenship

As health and social care practitioners it is therefore important that these principles are maintained for those individuals who access our services.

ADVOCACY

One form of intervention is advocacy. Advocacy can be defined as individual and group actions to effect change by writing and/or speaking in support of an issue outside of one's immediate group (Winkleby *et al.*, 2004). Advocacy serves as a mechanism to enable people to take control over their own lives. In a study of people with learning disabilities, Thomas and Woods (2003) demonstrate how advocacy services were used to enable participation and social inclusion.

The role of the health and social care practitioner in advocacy

For individuals who are disempowered through their circumstances of ill health or their social care needs, there may be a need for health and social care practitioners to intervene on their behalf and advocate or arrange for appropriate advocacy for them. It may be a case of a practitioner questioning a circumstance and taking a series of actions or steps that lead the circumstance towards what should be an appropriate outcome. Put simply, taking actions to change the 'what is' into a 'what should be'. However, advocacy does not always take place on an individual level as these five principal types of advocacy show (Rapaport *et al.*, 2005).

1. **Legal advocacy** – a broad range of methods and strategies using statutory frameworks and legislation (for example, the Human Rights Act 1988).

2. **Class advocacy** – this can be collective action, corporate or group action, and involves groups working together to promote the interests of the group, for example MIND, Help the Aged, the MS Society. Such groups can function in many ways, such as giving a voice to (misrepresented) citizen interests; mobilising citizens to participate in the democratic process or assisting in the development of better public policy through lobbying, for example (Young and Everritt, 2004).

3. **Self-advocacy** – a process of empowerment (see Chapter 8) used to encourage vulnerable and marginalised people to have a voice and to advocate for their own needs. This type of advocacy is central to anti-oppressive practice and fits with interventions designed to give people skills and opportunities to develop knowledge and confidence. It is fundamental to person-centred care and self-directed support.

4. **Peer advocacy** – people with similar experiences speak on behalf of others – examples would be local support projects and groups.

5. **Citizen advocacy** – vulnerable people or people with needs are linked to a volunteer who would advocate on their behalf (for example, befriending services for older people).

Activity

For each of the principal types of advocacy listed (Rapaport, 2005) can you think of a circumstance where this might be used?

- Legal advocacy.

- Class advocacy.

- Self-advocacy.

- Peer advocacy.

- Citizen advocacy.

One of the tensions for health and social care practitioners is being able to advocate for service users when resource constraints and other pressures may conflict with this role. There is no easy answer to this ethical dilemma. One way to address this is to signpost service users and carers to local advocacy services, so that they can access appropriate support. Thus, an awareness of the relevant services is an important tool in managing the ethical dilemmas that arise in a resource constrained care environment (McDonald, 2006).

SUMMARY

By introducing intervention within the ASPIRE framework of the care process this chapter has considered the nature and types of intervention in health and social care, discussing the reasons and rationale for undertaking specific interventions. The importance of using evidence-based interventions has been explored in terms of both cost-effectiveness and efficiency. Building on Chapter 5 it has re-emphasised the importance of working in partnership in order to enable intervention activity and has considered the role of advocacy for health and social care practitioners.

Reflection	
Identify at least three things that you have learned from this chapter.	1. 2. 3.
How do you plan to use this knowledge within care practice?	1. 2. 3.
How will you evaluate the effectiveness of your plan?	1. 2. 3.
What further knowledge and evidence do you need?	1. 2. 3.

FURTHER READING

Aveyard, H. and Sharp, P. (2009) *A Beginner's Guide to Evidence-Based Practice in Health and Social Care*. Buckingham: Open University Press

This book is for anyone who has ever wondered what evidence-based practice is or how to relate it to practice. It presents the topic in a simple, easy to understand way, enabling those unfamiliar with evidence-based practice to apply the concept to their practice and learning. Using everyday language, this book provides a step by step guide to what we mean by evidence-based practice and how to apply it. It also:

- provides an easy to follow guide to searching for evidence;
- explains how to work out if the evidence is relevant or not;
- explores how evidence can be applied in the practice setting;
- outlines how evidence can be incorporated into your academic writing.

Donnelly, E., Parkinson, T. and Williams, B. (2009) *Understanding and Helping People in Crisis*. Exeter: Reflect Press

This book is a user friendly and accessible guide for all those who support people who are experiencing personal crisis. Aimed at both students and practitioners, it introduces the reader to the concept of crisis touching upon global perspectives, local emergencies and personal experiences. Also, as a means of illustrating common experiences, the book presents a new model of crisis. It reviews personal narratives that reflect a range of common crises encountered in ordinary lives. The narratives and case studies reviewed identify gender and cultural influences alongside family, home and relationships as well as the impact that outside agencies, economics and occupation have on an individual at a time of crisis. It explores crisis theory – psychoanalytical theories, mental health, coping mechanisms and a transactional analysis perspective are explored, as well as cognitive and behavioural understandings of what happens to individuals when a crisis situation occurs – and offers an overview of crisis interventions. This discussion is enhanced through the detail of practical skills that have proved to be helpful in supporting people in crisis. Finally it reviews the potential outcomes for crisis. Positive and negative crisis resolutions, potential for recovery and change are explored and personal narratives are revisited. The final section includes detail regarding the more serious outcomes of crisis including post-traumatic stress disorder, mental illness, and the potential for suicide.

Hayes, S. and Llewellyn, A. (2008) *Fundamentals of Nursing Care: A Textbook for Students of Nursing and Healthcare*. Exeter: Reflect Press

Although care and the process of caring have been a fundamental part of nursing theories and paradigms for many years, there are an increasing number of anecdotal and media stories as well as academic debates that question the extent to which caring is satisfactorily carried out. *Fundamentals of Nursing Care* is a foundation level pre-registration text that aims to actively address this issue as it focuses on the fundamental principles of caring. The book covers topics such as: interpersonal issues; self and the therapeutic relationship; lay-professional conflicts; user articulation and the caring process; dignity and care; cultural competence and the process of care. The book is set out as a workbook, using narratives that are related to the NMC Essential Skills Clusters. Case studies are used to illustrate key points, and the book has been carefully designed to allow for critical incident analysis and enquiry-based and problem-based learning and reflection. Questions and activities encourage students to deconstruct practice and examine how to further develop competencies. There are also suggestions for additional reading throughout the book in order to support independent learning and enquiry.

Lindsay, T. (Ed) (2009) *Social Work Intervention* (Transforming Social Work Practice). Exeter: Learning Matters

Social workers (and health care workers) need to have a sound working knowledge of a range of ways of working with the people who use their services. They also need to be able to apply and integrate this knowledge in practice, to critically evaluate different methods and to choose the most effective in any particular set of circumstances This book provides a hands-on guide to the most common methods of helping social work service users and of dealing with some difficult situations. The authors set each method in its historical and theoretical context before explaining the method itself in easy to understand language. Case studies accompany and illustrate each method and the reader is invited to engage in a number of exercises and activities to consolidate learning.

Chapter 7

Evaluation and Review:

Evaluating Effective Care Delivery for Individuals, Services and Society

---

This chapter covers the following key issues:

- the evaluation and review of health and social care;
- quality drivers for contemporary health and social care policy;
- theory and models of quality assurance;
- the tools of quality assurance:

  - professionalism and professional standards;
  - regulation and monitoring;
  - the implementation of evidence-based practice in everyday working practice;
  - standard setting and benchmarking;
  - audit;
  - critical incident reporting and safety bulletin reporting;
  - reflective practice;
  - patient surveys and feedback.

By the end of this chapter you should be able to:

- understand the importance of evaluation and reviewing care at individual and service level;
- explain why it is important that health and social care is quality assured;
- discuss the tools and techniques that health and social care practitioners use to evaluate and review practice and services.

This chapter matches to the following National Occupational Standards and Essential Skills Clusters:

- ESC 1.vii Uses professional support structures to learn from experience and makes appropriate adjustments;
- ESC 12 Respond appropriately to feedback from patients/ clients, the public and a wide range of sources as a vehicle for learning and development;
- ESC 14.4 Reflects on own practice and discusses issues with other members of the team to enhance learning.
- NOS 6.4 Review the effectiveness of the plans with the people involved;
- NOS 13.3 Plan, monitor and review outcomes and actions to minimise stress and risk;
- NOS 14.3 Monitor and evaluate the effectiveness of your programme of work in meeting the organisational requirements and needs of individuals, families, carers, groups and communities;
- NOS 19.4 Critically reflect upon your own practice and performance using supervision and support systems.

INTRODUCTION

The final stage of the care process, as described by Sutton (1999), is review and evaluation. As stated, however, the process is cyclical and continuous, as review and evaluation may lead on to further assessment, starting the process again. Evaluation is not a one-off activity, but is ongoing. It is a process in which needs are continuously assessed and re-assessed according to ongoing evaluation.

Following current policy drivers, health and social care organisations are busy with efforts to improve the quality of care on a number of fronts (Walburg *et al.* 2006). Evaluating the effectiveness of care delivery for individuals, specific services and for society as a whole is important on a number of levels. Providing evidence-based interventions on both an individual and population level is about using the right care interventions on the right individual, but national drivers for the improvement of care delivery on both a service and national level also exist. This started prior to New Labour's period of office with the publication of the White Paper *Working for Patients* (DH, 1989b) but was continued in the *NHS Plan*

(DH, 2000a). These drivers are about quality, efficiency and effectiveness as well as safety and preventing health and social care disasters.

When Labour entered government in 1997 they published a policy called the *New NHS: Modern and Dependable* stating that

> The new NHS will have quality at its heart. Without it there is unfairness. Every patient who is treated in the NHS wants to know that they can rely on receiving high quality care when they need it. Every part of the NHS, and everyone who works in it, should take responsibility for working to improve quality . . .
>
> (DH, 1997a: 3.2)

This was about shifting 'the focus on to quality of care so that excellence is guaranteed to all patients' and the underpinning financial necessity of a need to 'improve efficiency so that every pound in the NHS is spent to maximise the care for patients' (DH, 1998a). A number of policy objectives followed, including *Clinical Governance: Quality in the New NHS* (NHS Executive, 1999) and, most recently, the result of the 'Darzi Review' – *High Quality Care for All* (DH, 2008d), all of which mandate professionals working in the NHS to improve clinical behaviours in order to improve outcomes for clinical practice and mandate services to improve the overall quality.

The Audit Commission is an independent body charged with ensuring that public money is spent economically, efficiently and effectively. In 2002 a system of Comprehensive Performance Assessment was introduced to monitor the performance of local councils and the effectiveness of their service provision. Under the Care Standards Act (DH, 2002d) a Performance Assessment Framework (PAF) was introduced to monitor the performance of all councils with social service responsibilities, with the Commission for Social Care Inspectorate (CSCI) being responsible for social care inspection (this has now joined with the health inspectorate, to become the Care Quality Commission (CQC) – see below). Social care monitoring and evaluation is conducted according to Performance Indicators (PIs) in the following areas:

- national priorities and strategic objectives;
- cost and efficiency;
- effectiveness of service delivery and outcomes;
- quality of services for users and carers;
- fair access to services.

THE PURPOSE OF EVALUATION

Evaluation simply means assessing the value of something and this raises an interesting question – value in terms of what? (Brophy *et al.*, 2008). This is dependent of course on who carries out the evaluation and why it is being carried out. Within health and social care, evaluation will normally be carried out to answer the question of whether the intervention has worked and whether the cost (financial or personal) was worth it. The difficulty is that, depending on who is concerned with the evaluation (the individual service user, the practitioner, the service provider or those who commission (pay for) the service), the question of 'is it worth it?' may have different answers.

> ## Activity
>
> Use the BBC news website (**www.bbc.co.uk**) to investigate the case regarding a Court of Appeal for Ms Rogers to access the drug Herceptin through the NHS as a pharmaceutical intervention for breast cancer (see **http://news.bbc.co.uk/1/hi/health/4684852.stm**).
>
> 1. Whose different perspectives in terms of evaluating the use of this drug were reported and how did they differ, before the ruling to allow Ms Rogers to receive the drug?

Importantly though, evaluations should be systematic, both in terms of the process and reporting. This means that they are carried out in a way that allows other people to follow the same process and understand how it was written up and how the results of the evaluation have been analysed (Brophy *et al.*, 2008).

Evaluating individual care

For individual service user interventions, care evaluation is about reviewing the effectiveness of care and serves two purposes (Hogston, 2007). First, the health or social care practitioner can ascertain whether the desired outcomes for the client have been achieved and, second, evaluation acts as an opportunity to review the entire process and determine whether the assessment was accurate and complete, any diagnostic element was correct, the goals of the intervention were realistic and achievable, and the resulting process of implementation was successful. Of course, the service user or care recipient is not a silent partner in this process, in the same way as they are not passive recipients of care. This means that health and social care practitioners must ensure that, as with every stage of ASPIRE, the voice of the service user is heard at the evaluation and review stage (see Chapter 5).

Answering a series of questions about each stage of the care process can assist with the review of care that is given at an individual level. Hogston (2007) suggests a number of questions (see Table 25), which were formulated to think about nursing care, but can also be adapted to review social care interventions.

---

1. Have the short-term goals been met?

2. If so, has the diagnosis or 'problem' been resolved so that it no longer needs to be addressed?

3. If the answer is no, then why have the care goals not been met? Did they meet the MACROS criteria (see page 138)?

4. Was the planned care intervention realistic, explicit, evidence-based, prioritised, involved and goal-centred (REEPIG)?

5. Was the method of intervention appropriate?

6. Was there effective communication within and between the care team?

7. Was the client satisfied with their care?

Table 25 Reviewing the nursing care plan (adapted from Hogston, 2007)

The GSCC Code of Practice for Social Care Employees (GSCC, 2002) is clear that social care practitioners have a duty to promote best practice, to keep up-to-date and to improve their own quality of work to maintain standards of care. For social workers, this is a pre-requisite for re-registration, so continuing professional development is an important part of the process of quality monitoring and enhancement.

Quality assurance of services

Much of the quality of care experienced by the individual service user is dependent on factors that are broader than the individual practitioner who is implementing a plan for the assessed care needs. Quality assurance refers to planned and systematic processes that try to provide confidence in an activity or intervention, or in a service or organisation's suitability for its intended purpose. Quality assurance activities aim to ensure that the services will meet requirements in a systematic, reliable way (Hayes and Llewellyn, 2008), and are a major component of current national policy (see Chapters 2 and 3).

Structure, process and outcome

Donabedian (1966) describes a model of quality assurance for the evaluation of health care, which can also be applied within the social care setting, and describes three approaches to specifying and measuring quality: structure, process and outcome. All three are considered equally important in measuring the quality of care provided by an organisation. They are complementary and they should be used collectively to monitor quality of care.

- **Structure** refers to human and physical resources and can include staff and policy.

- **Process** refers to the methods of working so may include the procedures for allocating resources or implementing guidelines.

- **Outcomes** refer to the effect of both the structure and the process, the result of a number of individual 'outputs'. The outcome relating to a clinical guideline being introduced, for example, would be improved patient care with improved clinical outcomes (Hayes and Llewellyn, 2008).

Huycke and All (2000) offer a simplistic way of looking at this by adding to the perspective of patients the perspectives of providers, payers and public. Hayes and Llewellyn (2008) interpret this model for the quality of health care provision as shown in Table 26.

Activity

1. Reflect on your last encounter with a service user.
2. Now consider how that care encounter has been quality assured from the perspectives of:

- Providers;
- Payers;
- Public;
- Patients.

Perspective	Focus
Providers (For example, health and social care organisations.)	The process and outcomes of care, including having the knowledge to deliver care and achieving the required health and social care outcomes (for example, meeting waiting list targets or having multi-agency protection policies).
Payers (For example, the general public in terms of taxpayers or private insurance.)	Affordability and access to care according to need.
Public	Standards and regulation set by the government (using the Health Care Commission's *Standards for Better Health* (DH, 2004e) or the *Performance Assessment Framework* for social services).
Patients	Subjective view of the quality of care.

Table 26 Model of quality perspectives (adapted from Hayes and Llewellyn, 2008)

The Balanced Scorecard approach

Another approach to quality assurance often used to evaluate whole organisations is the Balanced Scorecard (Kaplan and Norton, 1996). This involves the grouping of performance measures in general categories (perspectives) and is believed to aid organisations in the gathering and selection of the appropriate performance measures, thus contributing to Quality Assurance. Four general perspectives have been proposed by the Balanced Scorecard:

1. Financial perspective;
2. Customer perspective;
3. Internal process perspective;
4. Innovation and learning perspective.

The financial perspective within health and social care services may be one of remaining within budget and the questions that therefore need to be asked are about affordability and sustainability of interventions. The customer or service user perspective describes the satisfaction of the service user who receives the services. The internal process perspective is concerned with the processes that create and deliver the services, and considers all the activities and key processes required in order for the company or organisation to excel at providing the service effectively. The innovation and learning perspective focuses on the skills and capabilities that are required to deliver the required services. This is about the people who work within the services and asks whether they are trained and educated to do the job required of them, and whether the information systems are effective in enabling the organisations to keep up-to-date and informed (Kaplan and Norton, 1996).

Activity

Look at a Balanced Scorecard for one of the following: the GP Practice you are registered with, a local meals-on-wheels service, a home care service, or your local corner shop.

1. How might that service ensure quality performance in relation to the:

- financial perspective?
- customer perspective?
- internal process perspective?
- innovation and learning perspective?

THE TOOLBOX OF QUALITY ASSURANCE METHODS AND APPROACHES

Further tools of quality assurance that relate specifically to health and social care services are:

- professionalism and professional standards;
- regulation and monitoring;
- the implementation of evidence-based practice in everyday working practice;
- standard setting and benchmarking;
- audit;
- critical incident reporting and safety bulletin reporting;
- reflective practice;
- service user and carer surveys and feedback.

Professional standards

Nursing and health care

The Nursing and Midwifery Council (NMC) replaced the United Kingdom Central Council (UKCC) in 2002 as the body charged with establishing and maintaining a register of nurses and midwives who may legally practice. The NMC is also responsible for setting standards for the assessment of those wishing to enter the register and stay on it – essentially the establishment of professional competency and proficiency. The NMC established a range of competencies in 2004 that nurses need to achieve in order to be admitted to the register, as determined by the context of their practice area. Thus:

> Applicants for entry to the nurses' part of the register must achieve the standards of proficiency in the practice of adult nursing, mental health nursing, learning disabilities nursing or children's nursing.
> (NMC, 2004)

There are 17 standards of proficiency, which nurses must demonstrate that they have achieved in order to be entered on to Level 1 of the register and therefore become eligible to practice. These standards are focused on the assessment, planning and implementation of nursing care within ethical, legal and policy frameworks and are related to *The Standards of Conduct, Performance and Ethics for Nurses and Midwives* (NMC, 2008). One of these standards states that nurses must 'provide a high standard of practice and care at all times'.

In addition the NMC has published *Essential Skill Clusters for Pre-registration Nursing Programmes* (2007), which established the standards of proficiency required for entry to branch programmes and at the point of entry to the register. These clusters relate to the provision of care, but focus on more specific achievement of learning outcomes in relation to:

- care, compassion and communication;
- organisational aspects of care;
- infection prevention and control;
- nutrition and fluid management;
- medicines management.

Professional standards for social work practice

The General Social Care Council is the body charged with setting the standards for social work practice and, in conjunction with the Department of Health (2002) and TOPSS, established National Occupational Standards (NOS) for practice that a social worker must achieve in order to progress through the levels of their course and be registered as a qualified practitioner. This function has since been taken over by Skills for Care and Development (**www.skillsforcare.org.uk**). These occupational standards focus on a wide range of skills and competencies required for practice and reflect the subject benchmarks established by the Quality Assurance Agency (QAA). They are regularly reviewed in order to keep abreast of contemporary changes within the dynamic health and social care environment and requirements for professional practice.

The standards reflect the key purpose and roles of social work, derived from the international definition of social work as:

> a profession which promotes social change, problem-solving in human relationships and the empowerment and liberation of people to enhance well-being. Utilising theories of human behaviour and social systems, social work intervenes at the points where people interact with their environments. Principles of human rights and social justice are fundamental to social work.
>
> (International Association of Schools of Social Work and the International Federation of Social Workers, 2001)

The following six key roles are identified as necessary to fulfil the purpose of social work according to this definition.

Key Role 1: Prepare for, and work with individuals, families, carers, groups and communities to assess their needs and circumstances.

Key Role 2: Plan, carry out, review and evaluate social work practice, with individuals, families, carers, groups, communities and other professionals.

Key Role 3: Support individuals to represent their needs, views and circumstances.

Key Role 4: Manage risk to individuals, families, carers, groups, communities, self and colleagues.

Key Role 5: Manage and be accountable, with supervision and support, for your own social work practice within your organisation.

Key Role 6: Demonstrate professional competence in social work practice.

Regulation and monitoring

Both health and social care organisations have been historically monitored to ensure quality of performance by central government. One element of this is scrutiny organisations that, while they are commissioned by central government, are independent of them. This monitoring has historically been separate and, most recently, has been conducted in health by the Healthcare Commission and in social care by the Commission for Social Care Inspection and Mental Health Act Commission. However, as part of the Government's policy to improve working across the health and social care interface, the Care Quality Commission (CQC) was established by the Health and Social Care Act 2008 (DH, 2008e). This organisation is now responsible for regulating the quality of health and social care, and also for looking after the interests of individuals detained under the Mental Health Act (DH, 2007d) (CQC, 2008).

As the needs of people who use social care and health services, carers and their families have changed over the last decade, responsibility for social care and health services has come together. We see this across the country at local level as healthcare providers and Local Authorities bring their services together.

Now the Care Quality Commission will be the first opportunity to bring these functions together under one independent regulator. This will bring huge benefits:

- Giving people using services, their carers and families one port of call for information on standards, safety and available provision.

- Bringing together the best inspection and regulation methods, combining intelligence systems and statistical analysis with on-the-ground inspection and the views and verdicts of people who use health and social care services and the staff that work in health and social care.

- Giving an independent, authoritative view on the contribution that care makes to preventing illness and promoting ongoing healthy, independent living and wellbeing.

Table 27 The Care Quality Commission **www.cqc.org.uk/about_us/why_a_new_commission.aspx** (downloaded 2.2.09)

The CQC is responsible for registering, reviewing and inspecting services and, where providers of services fail to meet the legal requirements of their registration, it has the legal powers to take action against them. The aim is therefore to enable services to improve by ensuring that essential quality and safety standards are met and, where shortcomings are identified, use enforcement powers to force organisations to improve their standards. Enforcement powers include the power to:

- issue a warning notice;
- impose, vary or remove conditions;
- issue a penalty notice in lieu of prosecution;
- suspend registration;
- cancel registration;
- prosecute organisations for specified offences.

(CQC, 2008)

Implementing EBP in practice

Guidelines, clinical or non-clinical, are documents that guide decisions within services, based on the examination of current evidence and best practice. They summarise the consensus regarding specific interventions as well as some of the practical issues involved with their implementation. They address important questions related to clinical and non-clinical practice and identify all possible options and outcomes, sometimes following decision trees or algorithms which point to decision points and possible courses of action. Guidelines are important in setting the standards for care interventions in order to improve the quality of care, but also to enable equity of provision and ensure that the most effective and efficient treatments are used.

In 1999 the National Institute for Health and Clinical Excellence (NICE) was created as an independent organisation to provide national guidance on the promotion of good health and the prevention and treatment of ill health. NICE produces guidance in three areas of health:

1. **public health** – guidance on the promotion of good health and the prevention of ill health for those working in the NHS, Local Authorities and the wider public and voluntary sector.

2. **health technologies** – guidance on the use of new and existing medicines, treatments and procedures within the NHS.

3. **clinical practice** – guidance on the appropriate treatment and care of people with specific diseases and conditions within the NHS.

(NICE, 2008)

NICE carries out assessments of the most appropriate practice, taking into account both patient outcomes and the financial impact using the concept of Quality Adjusted Life Years (QALYs). Guideline Development Groups consist of medical professionals, representatives of patient and carer groups and technical experts who work together to assess the evidence base and best practice and, after a consultation period, issue guidance to the NHS.

Activity

When considering interventions for behaviour change visit the NICE website and search for relevant guidance.

The Social Care Institute for Excellence (SCIE) is a charitable organisation funded by the Department of Health, which identifies and disseminates knowledge about good practice to social care organisations. The aim is to provide knowledge and information to the diverse workforce in the social care field, as well as supporting developments in the transformation of care services to provide a more personalised service for users and carers. In addition, SCIE provides support, knowledge and information to service users and carers themselves:

> We recognise the central role of people who use services, children, young people, their families and their carers, and we aim to ensure their experience and expertise is reflected in all aspects of our work.
>
> (www.scie.org.uk)

Benchmarking and standard setting

Benchmarking is the process of comparing the quality of what one organisation or service does against what another organisation or service does, with the result giving evidence as to whether changes or improvements need to be made. National Guidelines set criteria for benchmarking but, in addition to this, *The Essence of Care* was launched in 2001 by the Modernisation Agency of the NHS with the aim of establishing benchmarks for clinical governance to help health care practitioners to adopt a patient-focused and structured approach to sharing and comparing practice (Hayes and Llewellyn, 2008).

Benchmarks have been published on:

- continence and bladder and bowel care;
- personal and oral hygiene;
- food and nutrition;
- pressure ulcers;
- privacy and dignity;
- record keeping;
- safety of clients with mental health needs in acute mental health and general hospital settings;
- principles of self-care;
- promoting health (added in 2006);
- care environment (added in 2007).

Table 28 *The Essence of Care* benchmarks (DH, 2001e, 2006d and 2007e)

Health care practitioners have worked with care recipients to identify best practice and to develop plans for improving quality of care, relevant to all health and social care settings. The benchmarks are therefore presented in generic format, so that they can be used in primary, secondary or tertiary care settings and with a range of user and carer groups. Initially eight benchmarks were established, but further benchmarks were added later in response to feedback from practitioners and service users. Benchmarks are used in practice as standards against which to undertake quality audits.

The audit cycle

Audit is at the heart of quality improvement as it can be used as a tool to review and improve all services by:

- providing the mechanisms for reviewing the quality of everyday care;
- building on a long history of health care professionals reviewing case notes and seeking ways to serve their patients better;
- addressing quality issues systematically and explicitly, providing reliable information;
- confirming the quality of services and highlighting the need for improvement.

(Adapted from NICE, 2002)

Clinical audit is a quality improvement process that seeks to improve patient care and outcomes through systematic review of care against explicit criteria and the implementation of change. Aspects of the structure, processes, and outcomes of care are selected and systematically evaluated against explicit criteria. Where indicated, changes are implemented at an individual, team, or service level and further monitoring is used to confirm improvement in healthcare delivery.

Clinical audit can be described as a cycle or a spiral. Within the cycle there are stages that follow a systematic process of establishing best practice, measuring care against criteria, taking action to improve care, and monitoring to sustain improvement. The spiral suggests that as the process continues, each cycle aspires to a higher level of quality.

Table 29 What is clinical audit? (NICE, 2002)

The following (Figure 16) is an example of the audit cycle (**www. qualityinoptometry.co.uk**).

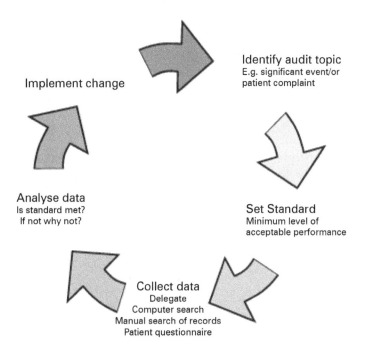

Figure 16 The audit cycle

Activity

Visit *The Essence of Care* website and examine one of the benchmarks. Design an audit to determine the quality of a service against the benchmark that you have identified.

Critical incident analysis and service user safety

It is recognised that critical incidents or adverse care events cannot be eliminated from complex modern health and social care, and learning from such events to improve future service user safety has been an important step in recent years. The identification of such critical incidents should result in an audit being undertaken so that this learning will take place. Critical incidents are an observable activity where there is sufficient information to make inferences or predictions about the person who is carrying out the act, the purpose or intention of the act and, importantly, the effects of the act (Flanagan, 1954). Furthermore, it has been recognised that there is a need to collect and analyse accurate data on adverse health care events and in 2000 the Department of Health published its Paper *Organisation with a Memory* to formalise this process (DH, 2000d). This has led to a national system emphasising the need to collect and analyse accurate data on adverse health care events. The format for doing so is based on the process of:

- gathering information on the root cause of the incident (i.e. identify the factors that led to the incident/hazard occurring);
- learning from it (i.e. study it and consult widely);
- acting to prevent it happening again (identify interventions which may prevent reoccurrence) and so . . .
- preventing or reducing risk.

Case study

Administration of Vinca alkaloids such as vincristine (drugs used in chemotherapy treatments for cancer patients) by the spinal route (intrathecally), rather than intravenously, invariably causes death or neurological damage. This catastrophic clinical error has arisen because of confusion of drugs with a cytotoxic agent intended to be given intrathecally (usually methotrexate). Five such incidents have occurred in NHS hospitals in the past decade, representing an estimated rate of about three per 100 000 intrathecal chemotherapy treatments.

www.dh.gov.uk/en/Publicationsandstatistics/Publications/ PublicationsPolicyAndGuidance/DH_4065044

Organisation with a Memory (2000d) set a target regarding this error:

'By 2001, reduce to zero the number of patients dying or being paralysed by mal-administered spinal injections.'

Activity

When the incident was investigated:

1. What information on the root cause of the incident was found?
2. What was learnt from it?
3. What action was taken to prevent it happening again?
4. Was risk reduced?

The National Patient Safety Agency, established in 2001, has the responsibility of improving the safety and quality of patient care through reporting, analysing, and disseminating the lessons of adverse events and 'near misses' involving NHS patients.

Serious case reviews

Serious case reviews are undertaken to evaluate a critical incident when a child has died (including suicide), and when abuse or neglect is either known to be or is suspected to be a factor in that death. They may also be carried out where:

- a child sustains a potentially life-threatening injury or serious and permanent impairment of health and development through abuse or neglect;
- a child has been subjected to particularly serious sexual abuse;

- a parent has been murdered and a homicide review is being initiated;
- a child has been killed by a parent with a mental illness;
- or the case gives rise to concerns about inter-agency working to protect children from harm.

The nature of serious case reviews is set out in Chapter 8 of the document *Working Together to Safeguard Children* (DH, 2006b) (**www.everychildmatters.gov.uk/workingtogether**). The purpose of serious case reviews is to:

- establish whether there are lessons to be learned from the case about the way in which local professionals and agencies work together to safeguard and promote the welfare of children;
- identify clearly what those lessons are, how they will be acted on, and what is expected to change as a result;
- and, consequentially, to improve inter-agency working and better safeguard and promote the welfare of children.

Serious case reviews may also be undertaken where an adult has died and there is suspicion or evidence of neglect or abuse, as in the case of Steven Hoskin. Mr Hoskin was a 39-year-old man with learning disabilities who was subjected to systematic abuse by carers, who hauled him around his bed-sit with a dog collar, burned him with cigarettes and eventually made him cling to a viaduct, where he fell to his death after being kicked in the face and having his hands stamped on. Although Steven Hoskin was known to social services, insufficient action was taken to safeguard him from this abuse.

Activity

Read the summary of the serious case review into Steven Hoskin's death at **http://www.cornwall.gov.uk/m_pdf/a_e_SCR_Executive_Summary1_Dec_2007_.pdf**

What lessons can be learned to improve future practice?

In addition to the National Patient Safety Agency, the Medicines and Healthcare products Regulatory Agency (MHRA) was created and is the government agency that is responsible for ensuring that medicines and medical devices work, and are acceptably safe.

Activity

The MHRA monitors safety and the quality standards of medicines and medical devices in several ways. For example:

Regular inspections to ensure good and safe practice in;

- manufacturers and suppliers of medicines and medical devices,
- medicines distribution and storage,
- clinical trials,
- clinical inspecting systems for devices,
- laboratories testing medicines,
- auditing Notified Bodies,
- blood establishments.

**www.mhra.gov.uk/Safetyinformation/
Howwemonitorthesafetyofproducts/index.htm**

Visit the MHRA website and investigate in what other ways they contribute to the safety of service users.

Critical incident analysis

However, it is not only major averse health and social care events that impact on the care that service users receive and it is therefore important that practitioners individually reflect on the care they provide through critical incident analysis. This involves reflecting on either good or bad practice to give insight into that practice. It is not solely concerned with the identification of ineffective or incompetent practice (Rich and Parker, 1995) as learning can be achieved though the identification of and reflection on actions that have had positive outcomes for the care recipient. The use of critical incident analysis as a tool to improve care giving depends on the ability of individuals to reflect upon and question practice and, therefore, the ability of the caregiver to recognise either a dissonance between the care given and the required outcome for the care recipient or, conversely, to recognise why good outcomes were achieved (Hayes and Llewellyn, 2008).

Reflective practice

Reflective practice is a process that must be undertaken by all registered nurses, both personally and through the process of clinical supervision

(UKCC, 1996), and by social workers as part of their ongoing learning (NOS Key Role 5). The process of reflective practice is being used by different professional groups, with the aim of improving care through changing practice.

However, reflection is not new. Dewey's appraisal of reflective thought as that which results from an event in life that provokes or arouses a state of perplexity or uncertainty and leads the individual to search for possible explanations or solutions (Dewey, 1933 in Quinn, 2000) can be applied throughout the human experience. It could be argued to be what makes us human. Human agents design actions to achieve certain ends and monitor ongoing action and its consequence to assess its effectiveness (Greenwood, 1998). Boud, Keough and Walker (1985, p. 19) define reflection as:

> Those intellectual and affective activities in which individuals engage to explore their experiences in order to lead to new understandings and appreciations.

Schon (1978, in Quinn, 2000) focused on the relationship between academic knowledge and professional competence. He describes reflection in action, which is inherent in a current action, and reflection on action, which involves retrospection on the experience, and he identified that there is a need to narrow the gap between theory and practice.

There is, though, a difference between knowledge and 'knowing' and a distinction between explicit knowledge and tacit knowledge. Explicit knowledge presented as fact only has relevance on an individual basis if it informs and fits with 'knowing' – that is the tacit knowledge that each of us possesses, based on years of experience, which is described by some as 'gut instinct' (Greener, 2004). It is about the ways in which we 'know'. That is knowing 'how to do' (practice knowledge) or knowing 'that' (acquired information) (Ryle, 1949 in Woodman *et al.*, 2002). Carper's model of 'fundamental patterns of knowing' (1978) describes the various kinds of knowing about practice, which include tacit elements and also a recognition of the personal meaning that underpins learning and knowledge for each individual. The patterns are:

- **empirical** – factual and verifiable;
- **aesthetic** – the subjective element, honed by experience;
- **personal** – aimed at actualising authentic personal relationships between the practitioner and their patient client;

- **ethical** – acknowledgement that all actions are subject to the value of right and wrong.

Johns (2004) incorporated Carper's (1978) 'ways of knowing' into a model of reflection to allow the practitioner to appreciate personal, ethical and empirical influences on the experience, thereby framing learning through reflection. Johns describes (believing definition impels authority) reflection as:

> A fusion of sensing, perceiving and intuitive thinking related to a specific experience to develop insights into self and practice. It is a vision-driven process, concerned with taking action towards knowing and realising desirable practice.
>
> (Johns, 2004, pp. 2–3)

Gibbs' (1988) reflective cycle clearly demonstrates the cyclical and continual process of reflection.

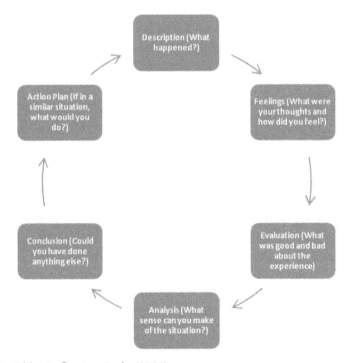

Figure 17 Gibbs' Reflective Cycle (1988)

Service user and carer surveys and feedback

Service user and carer satisfaction is another factor taken into consideration when judging quality of care, and service user and carer surveys and feedback are being increasingly used in health and social care services. Organisations can gather user feedback in a variety of ways including surveys, audits, comments and complaints, focus groups and interviews (Picker Institute, 2009). Health and social care organisations are mandated to undertake user surveys and actively seek feedback. By constantly and systematically surveying care, a detailed picture of the experience of services users is drawn. National surveys are valuable as they allow local organisations to compare their performance to that of similar organisations across the country. It also means that it is possible to identify the things that really matter to service users. The Picker Institute, for example, who are commissioned to survey the National Health Service, have found that the things that are most important to service users are:

- fast and reliable health advice;
- effective treatments delivered by trusted professionals;
- participation in decisions and respect for preferences;
- clear, comprehensive information and support for self-care;
- attention to physical and environmental needs;
- emotional support, empathy and respect;
- involvement of, and support for family and carers;
- continuity of care and smooth transitions.

(Picker Institute, 2009)

In addition to service user and carer surveys, Patient Reported Outcome Measures (PROMs) are going to be collected routinely as a result of the policy *High Quality Care for All* set out by Lord Darzi (DH, 2008d). PROMs is a method of collecting information on the quality of clinical care as reported by service users themselves. Service users answer the same set of questions on their quality of life before and after an operation and the comparable data is then used to calculate a numerical value for the improvement to their health. The focus for this approach will start with all licensed providers of hip replacements, groin hernia and varicose vein surgery (DH, 2009g).

While a surgeon may judge a hip replacement successful because the procedure has been performed perfectly on the day, the patient will rightly disagree if they are still in pain and continue to have a poor quality of life six months down the line.

The beauty of PROMs is that it measures the success of operations as reported by patients themselves. This programme is the first of its kind in the world and the information collected will empower patients to choose a hospital that achieves the best results for the operation they need.

It will also strengthen commissioning across the NHS by offering PCTs the evidence they need to buy the best services based on patient experiences. What's more, routine collection of PROMs will enable clinical teams to benchmark their performance and research the success of different treatment options.

(DH, 2009g)

Activity

Think of a recent encounter with a service user involving some kind of intervention. How would the PROM work in that scenario?

SUMMARY

This chapter focused on the evaluation and review stage of ASPIRE. It is essential that health and social care practitioners understand the importance of evaluating health and social care at individual service user level, organisational level and national level. There are many contemporary policy drivers and a plethora of tools and techniques that can be used in order to ensure that care is effectively quality assured and evaluated.

Reflection	
Identify at least three things that you have learned from this chapter.	1. 2. 3.
How do you plan to use this knowledge within care practice?	1. 2. 3.
How will you evaluate the effectiveness of your plan?	1. 2. 3.
What further knowledge and evidence do you need?	1. 2. 3.

FURTHER READING

Brophy, S., Snooks, H. and Griffiths L.J. (2008) *Small-Scale Evaluation in Health: A Practical Guide*. London: Sage

Setting out the basics of designing, conducting and analysing an evaluation study in health care, the authors take a practical approach, assuming no previous knowledge or experience of evaluation. All the basics are covered, including: how to plan an evaluation; research governance and ethics; understanding data; interpreting findings; writing a report. Case studies are included throughout to demonstrate evaluation in action, and self learning courses give the reader an opportunity to develop their skills further in the methods and analysis involved in evaluation.

Gomm, R. and Davies, C. (2000). *Using Evidence in Health and Social Care*. Buckingham: Open University Press

This wide-ranging text on research methods in health and social care introduces readers to different kinds of evidence and helps them to evaluate the unique contributions of each. It acknowledges the variety of contexts in which practitioners work and the challenges of putting research into practice. The book introduces readers to research of different kinds – the randomised controlled trial, the survey, qualitative research and action research – and highlights the underlying logic and value of each. It also addresses economic appraisal and ethical issues in research. The text goes on to consider how there can be a much more active and dynamic interplay between practice and research, and using examples from health and social care shows that applying evidence is a complex process requiring the active participation of those on the receiving end.

Chapter 8

Challenges for the Future of Health and Social Care

This chapter covers the following key issues:

- definitions of power and the context within which power operates;
- factors that impact on collaborative and partnership working;
- the use of assistive technologies for independent living.

By the end of this chapter you should be able to:

- explain how issues of power might impact on the ASPIRE process;
- examine issues that impact on user involvement in decision-making processes in health and social care;
- discuss arguments about skill mix in health and social care and the relationship to processes of quality and regulation.

This chapter matches to the following National Occupational Standards and Essential Skills Clusters:

- ESC 1.xiv Uses professional support structures to develop self-awareness, challenge own prejudices and enable professional relationships, so that care is delivered without compromise;
- ESC 4.vii Is proactive in promoting care environments that are culturally sensitive and free from discrimination, harassment and exploitations;
- ESC 4.viii Manages challenging situations effectively;
- ESC 11.x Challenges practices that do not safeguard those requiring support and protection.
- NOS 12.2 Balance the rights and responsibilities of individuals, families, carers, groups and communities with associated risk;

- NOS 17.4 Deal constructively with disagreements and conflicts within relationships;
- NOS 20.1 Identify and assess issues, dilemmas and conflicts that might affect your practice;
- NOS 20.2 Devise strategies to deal with ethical issues, dilemmas and conflicts.

INTRODUCTION

The discussions throughout the preceding chapters have demonstrated that adult health and social care services are witnessing a period of radical transformation, with a move away from a welfarist model of service delivery, to person-centred care, based on individual assessment of needs and the provision of services to promote independent living wherever possible. Similarly, the emphasis in children's health and social care provision is on empowerment and rights, alongside ensuring that vulnerable children are safeguarded from abuse and harm.

The Green Paper *Shaping the Future of Care Together* (DH, 2009f) identifies six key values and policy imperatives for transforming adult social care (see Figure 18). While there is evidence of good practice in relation to all of these key areas throughout the UK, there is also evidence that this is patchy, and there is a need for sharing best practice to ensure that all people who are recipients of care services receive the most appropriate services for their needs.

> Ensuring older people, people with chronic conditions, disabled people and people with mental health problems have the best possible quality of life and the equality of independent living is fundamental to a socially just society.
>
> (DH, 2009f)

Assessment and good planning of care in conjunction with the service users and their carers is crucial to improving the quality of care for all, and requires a fundamental shift in attitudes to reflect this new focus on self-assessment and addressing needs as the recipients of services identify them. While these transformations offer positive ways of working and valuing people, they also pose a number of challenges for professionals working within health and social care, as well as for service users and their carers.

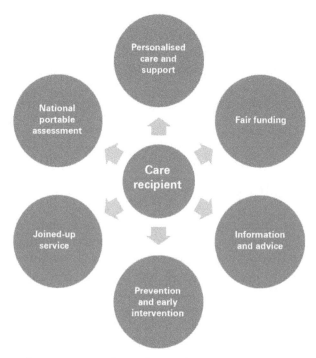

Figure 18 Key policy imperatives from *Shaping the Future of Care Together* (DH, 2009f)

As discussed throughout this book, user involvement and person-centred care remains a continuing policy priority in health and social care, but variations in service user involvement across service user groups as well as between different organisations and service providers remain. Achieving user involvement in health and social care decision-making, in both shaping their own health and social care needs and in the wider context of provision, continues to present a challenge for health and social care professionals. The challenge is to build on models of good practice so that there is true service user and carer involvement in decision-making, assessment and service provision, with true partnerships in care, rather than tokenistic involvement.

A second challenge for health and social care professionals stems from policies that aim to increase independent living and social inclusion. Since the 1990 National Health Service and Community Care Act, there has been an emphasis on maximising independent living in adult social care, and this has been further strengthened through the personalisation agenda and self-directed support. In addition, since 1997, the Labour Government emphasised the importance of tackling social exclusion, particularly among the most marginalised groups of adults and children in society. The Government launched the Social Exclusion Unit in 1997, with the purpose of creating cross-departmental policies to help the most disadvantaged in society. In 2002 the Office of the Deputy Prime Minister took on the responsibility of tackling social exclusion, and this remains a central focus of Government policy (**www.parliament.uk/ parliamentary_committees/odpm.cfm** (last accessed 25.1.10)).

Resource issues are also a constant challenge in a health and social care environment where demographic changes (see Chapters 2 and 3) and changing expectations are placing increasing demands on service providers. This is particularly pertinent in times of economic recession, with increased scrutiny of public expenditure in relation to statutory services, and it raises issues about the operation of the mixed economy of welfare and the effective and efficient use of both individual and organisational budgets. There are also challenges in terms of workforce development and the training, education, monitoring and regulation of service providers (including people paid as personal assistants within the personalisation and independent living agenda).

Radical transformation of health and social care services requires a cultural change in attitudes from both service users and carers, and professionals, with challenges to unequal power relationships as well as expectations about the way that services are developed and delivered. In addition, the emphasis on safeguarding vulnerable people has to be balanced against empowering people to make their own decisions and to take positive risks.

Globally, there has been a technological revolution throughout the latter half of the twentieth century and continuing into the twenty-first century (Macionis and Plummer, 2005), which has led to fundamental changes in societal organisation in every aspect of life, including health and social care provision. Technological developments offer new ways of working and can be positive in terms of new networking opportunities and developments in independent living, but offer challenges in relation to resources and partnership working.

All of these challenges are relevant to the ASPIRE process, as the transformations in ways of working with both adults and children require a fundamental shift in professional attitudes and the balance of power between professionals and service users and carers.

POWER

The concept of power is central to the challenges in assessing, planning, implementing and evaluating health and social care in the twenty-first century and underpins many of the issues outlined above. So what do we mean when we talk about power and how does this relate to health and social care practice? Power is a term that is frequently used in all walks of life but, as a theoretical concept, it is difficult to define. There is no single definition of power and it will mean different things in different social contexts, but it is useful to look at a number of different elements that are related to the concept of power.

Power is all around us and is a pervasive element of social relations, operating between individuals, as well as through social organisations, political groups and formal institutions (Gubbay, 1997). Therefore, when exploring power it is important to understand the social context that it operates in as well as the outcome of the actions.

Activity

1. Make a list of the ways in which power has been used within your life (when you have completed reading this chapter, go back to this list and think about any additions that you would make).
2. Think about the role of a health or social care practitioner when assessing the care needs of an individual.

   a) Who holds the power?
   b) What factors contribute to a power imbalance in health and social care?

Powerlessness and oppression

Power is an important concept in health and social care as individuals and groups that engage with services may be disadvantaged through disempowerment in a number of ways. The concept of oppression is related to power and serves to limit individuals' participation in the decision-making process. Oppression can be defined as a:

system of interrelated barriers and forces that reduce, immobilise and mould people who belong to a certain group in ways that effect their subordination to another group.

(Kendall, 1992)

The following groups, who are significant users of health and social care services, have been particularly powerless and oppressed in society:

- people with mental health problems;
- people with learning disabilities;
- people with physical disabilities;
- people with long-term conditions;
- children (especially looked-after children);
- older people;
- people who are homeless;
- ex-offenders.

(Thompson, 2007)

The concept of psychological or personal power can be used to further explore disempowerment and oppression. This affects the individual's ability to achieve their goals and to address their own needs or make their own decisions, and is related to the skills, attributes, roles and attitudes that the individual has (Thompson, 2007).

Skills

The exercising of power is affected by the individual's skills such as communication or assertiveness. The sociologist Bernstein (1975) developed a theory of socio-linguistics, exploring the relationship that individuals have to language and how this relates to the social structures of society and the social position of individuals in this structure. The impact of this can be illustrated through the research of Cartwright and O'Brien (1976), who found that people from higher social classes got more out of the doctor/patient consultation than people in lower social classes. They suggested that one reason for this was that these people spoke a similar language to the doctor in terms of culture and values and were therefore more easily able to initiate conversation and articulate their needs to achieve the outcomes that they wanted.

Activity

Think about the following words/phrases that health and social care practitioners might use:

'Take these suppositories and place one in your back passage every night.'
'Are you managing to feed yourself OK?'
'Do you drink enough?'
'How is your pain today?'

- Is the interpretation clear?
- What alternative interpretations might people put on these phrases?

Thus communication and the way people use language is an important aspect of power and disempowerment, and it impacts on the ways that people use health and social care services and the extent to which they feel empowered to make their own decisions and engage in the processes of care. For example, overlooking or misinterpreting communication with children can lead to them being excluded from the decision-making process or erroneous decisions being made (Jones, 2003), and effective communication with children is emphasised as a priority in professional education programmes for nurses and social workers. There is a growing body of research that explores ways of reaching people whose voices have not traditionally been heard (Sartain *et al.*, 2000; Killick and Allan, 2001; Goldsmith, 2002).

Attributes

The personal characteristics of an individual may affect their ability to exert power due to the ideological constructions of society. This means that through discourses and social reproduction (the ways that people talk about and accept situations as normal and are happy for that approach to continue), society constructs ideas about the relative value of different attributes, leading to the construction of dominant groups. For example, it is argued that Western societies are somatic societies, with a focus on the body and constructions of the normal/abnormal body and therefore the relative worth and value of the individual (Llewellyn *et al.*, 2008). Historically, people with disabilities or impairments were segregated into institutions as they were seen as abnormal (Barnes, 1991). This segregation contributed to a fear of the unknown and people with disabilities came to be seen as inferior and as people to be feared, leading to stereotyping and marginalisation. Similarly, in a society that places value on youth (Fischer, 1978), older people are stereotyped on the basis of their physical appearance and stereotypical assumptions are made about physical and mental deterioration, contributing to financial and social marginalisation (Featherstone and Hepworth, 1991). Therefore, the body is an important site of power and control and those who are devalued on the basis of physical attributes are marginalised and disempowered in social relations. This can be extended to the value placed on people in terms of perceived mental ability and stereotypical assumptions about individual's behaviour and participation (see, for example, Hazan (2000) for a discussion of stereotypical assumptions about older peoples' abilities and value). Also, a number of health conditions are stigmatised in society, which involves a process of social labelling leading to devaluing and negative attitudes (Moon and Gillespie, 1995).

Activity

When I applied for a job as a cleaner at a care home the manager called me and wanted to know more about my disability, which I'd declared. She pressed me so I said 'I'll be absolutely open with you. I've got a schizoaffective disorder and I hear the voices of people I knew.' There was complete silence on the phone. She didn't say a word. So I said 'Hello, are you still there?' All she said was 'I'll be in touch'. Anyway, a few days later, lo and behold, I received a rejection letter. To me her silence spoke volumes and I felt very discriminated against.

Extract from Department of Health (2006e) *Action on Stigma*

1. What stereotypes are apparent here?
2. What are the implications of this negative social labelling in terms of power?

The marginalisation and stigmatisation of people is related to disempowerment within the care processes, and health and social care professionals need to take this into account when engaging service users in the assessment and planning of care needs. Health and social care professionals also need to be aware of their own values and the influence that wider social issues may have in terms of stereotypical assumptions about service users' abilities and skills. A model of reflective practice and self-reflexivity is important in helping practitioners to critically reflect on their own value base and explore ways that this might impact on the ASPIRE process (see Chapter 7).

Roles

People have different roles in society and these roles are ranked hierarchically based on the social construction of value. This is partly related to attributes as discussed above, but also relates to dominant sets of ideas, where dominant groups are able to use power to perpetuate this hierarchical division to further their own advantage. Society is divided on class, gender and ethnic lines (Giddens, 2006) as well as constructions of age, sexuality and ability (Llewellyn *et al.*, 2008).

It should also be remembered that there may be crossover between these categories. For example, an older person may also be homeless or suffer from mental health problems. In addition, their degree of power may be further influenced by the social variables of class, gender, ethnicity and sexuality.

Activity

Consider the scenario where a nurse and a doctor disagree about the best way to treat a patient. What sort of factors in terms of their roles might influence the power dynamic here?

Attitudes

People's own attitudes can affect their ability to exert power and control over their own lives. Issues such as confidence, self-esteem and willingness to take risks are all important indicators of a person's attitude and ability to take control. Self-esteem can be influenced by a number of factors, including how we perceive ourselves and how others see and value us, and it is closely related to our levels of confidence (Thompson and Thompson, 2008). Inner resources and life cycle experiences are important contributors to people's attitudes and sense of power, but so too are the environments and structures within which those experiences are shaped. The social construction of dominant ideas may have a powerful impact on people as they come to internalise those dominant value systems and they may therefore see themselves as not having the ability to do something.

Power therefore can be seen as the ability to do something based on personal and psychological processes, but it is also related to wider social structures and institutional practices and power over other people. The development of a welfarist model of care (see Chapters 1 and 2) focused power in the hands of welfare professionals, who had the power to define needs, assess people's level of needs and plan and deliver interventions based on eligibility criteria and availability of services. Throughout the twentieth and twenty-first centuries there has been increased state involvement in family policy and Donzelot (1980) has argued that welfare professionals have been increasingly involved in the policing of the family. As agents of the state, he argues, health and social care professionals are involved in surveillance and protection of families, based on ideas of normalisation and moralisation, and thus they perpetuate dominant sets of values and morals.

Power is therefore a concept that applies to the influence that people are able to exert over others. This is sometimes referred to as ideological power (the extent to which individuals can influence dominant sets of ideas in society), or structural power (the extent to which individuals are empowered within the structures and institutions of society to exert control over others) (Gramsci, 1971). A good example of this is the power that the medical profession has had in the assessment of needs and the welfarist approach to assessing people for services as discussed in Chapter 1.

Power within organisations

Weber (1976) used the term rational-legal authority to describe the power that individuals have within organisations. Weber was interested in how complex organisations are structured to achieve their goals, and used the term 'bureaucracy' to describe an organisation that is structured according to hierarchical division of offices, with a top-down chain of command and a set of rules to govern behaviour and practices within the organisation. Those who hold higher positions in the hierarchy are seen to have legitimate power and authority by virtue of their position.

This theory remains relevant for understanding the way that complex organisations such as the NHS and Social Services are organised, and can be seen in new managerialist systems of organisation that have been implemented as part of the modernisation agenda in health and social care (Healy, 2000; Adams *et al.*, 2002). While bureaucracies may be seen as the epitome of rational-legal authority within institutions, they have also been criticised for the overemphasis on rules and procedures. For example, there have been criticisms that health and social care services have become too focused on achieving the targets and performance criteria to measure the performance of the organisation (Pollock and Talbot-Smith, 2006) at the expense of assessing the needs of individuals and providing a person-centred service. Parry-Jones and Soulsby (2001) have argued that needs-led assessment is difficult to pursue in practice, where practitioners continue to be gatekeepers to scarce resources. Hence, there may be more emphasis on the needs of the organisation than on the needs of the individual service user, with eligibility criteria being used as a way of rationing resources.

Power therefore operates at an organisational and structural level and this can impact on the care process. Power also operates at the level of individuals and is an important aspect of social relationships. As discussed in Chapter 4, differentials in power at this individual level can impact on the assessment process.

Activity

Breaching waiting lists.

There are a number of ways that priority for admission to hospital or eligibility for care services can be managed:

- first-come, first-served basis;
- assessment of clinical priority;
- ability to pay.

1. Which system fits best with Weber's concept of rational-legal authority?
2. What are the implications of these different systems for efficient management of welfare services?
3. Read the following article for a more detailed discussion of management of waiting lists.

Goddard, J. and Tavakoli, M. (2008) 'Efficiency and welfare implications of managed public sector hospital waiting lists'. *European Journal of Operational Research* 184 (2008) 778–792

Abstract

A queuing model for public health service waiting lists is developed, and the implications for patient welfare of different systems for managing the waiting list are analysed. If patients are admitted to hospital on a first-come, first-served basis, a welfare gain is achieved by moving from a system of implicit to one of explicit rationing of access to the waiting list. If individual waiting times and hospital admissions are dependent on clinical priority, a further welfare gain is achievable without the use of explicit rationing, by reallocating the total waiting time from the more towards the less seriously ill. On efficiency and welfare criteria, a maximum waiting time guarantee does not appear to be a desirable development.

The ways in which individuals may exercise power

1. Persuasion

An individual may be persuaded to do something by another person because of their superior status. Thus, within a hierarchical system of organisation, people who are seen to have authority by virtue of their superior position in the hierarchy can persuade subordinates of appropriate courses of action.

Activity

Tony works as a health care assistant in a care home. He has only been there for a couple of months and does not agree with the manager's practice of insisting that all the residents have a rest period straight after lunch. However, he goes along with the practice, as he feels uncomfortable about challenging the manager, particularly as all other staff seem happy to comply.

1. What elements of persuasion are apparent here?

2. People may be induced to behave in a certain way

For example, a service user may be induced to comply with a professional assessment of needs or plan of intervention for fear of being labelled unpopular (Stockwell, 1972) or not receiving any services.

3. Anticipated reaction

People may do or not do something in anticipation of a reaction from another person. People may therefore behave in a way that they would not otherwise have done in order to get the reaction that they want or feel is expected of them. For example, a person may appear grateful for a prescription when they actually have no intention of taking the pills, as they feel that this is what the doctor or nurse expects of them.

4. Disciplinary power

The normal workings of society constantly reaffirm and reproduce the existing power structures through registration, inspection, certification, surveillance and individuation. Thus, nurses and social workers have power by virtue of their registration as professionals and the certification of their knowledge base. This has impacted on the welfarist model of assessing people for services as discussed in Chapters 1 and 2.

5. Habituation

This is where the person is so used to complying that it is done automatically. An example of this is where a person becomes institutionalised, with loss of liberty and freedom and an emphasis on organisational priorities rather than individual needs. King and Raynes (1968) identify four features of an institution: depersonalisation; social distance between staff and residents; block activities, where activities are rigidly organised at a group level providing little opportunity for individuals to state their preferences; a lack of variety in daily routine. Hospitals, care homes and group homes may all be examples of institutions, but service users may also become institutionalised within their own homes where organisational processes limit their freedoms.

Power as a benefit to service users

Power then can affect the interpersonal relationship and the way in which the ASPIRE process operates. However, power can also be used to provide benefits for service users. We can use the term 'power with' to explore the concept of power within society. 'Power with' refers to the power derived from working together in partnership or collaboratively with other individuals (see Chapter 5).

> The more we network the more powerful we can become and the more united our voice will be. We will be stronger. To develop a strong voice is important and from other groups we must learn to develop our own networks.
>
> (Branfield and Beresford, 2006)

Activity

Read the following extract:

Once in the lounge patients had to be removed again at regular intervals to be reordered or taken to the toilet. Then they went to lunch, back to bed for two hours, up again for late tea, to the toilet, into dinner, to the toilet, to the lounge, to the toilet and finally to bed. During the night, auxiliaries undertook two-hourly rounds in which each patient was checked and their body ordered as necessary.

(Lee-Treweek, 1997: 54)

1. In what ways are the patients in this extract institutionalised?
2. In what ways do staff exercise power?
3. How are the patients disempowered?
4. What could be done differently so that residents could exert more power?

This power can be seen in the development of user and carer groups who have become involved in decision-making at all levels of health and social care delivery.

USER INVOLVEMENT IN HEALTH AND SOCIAL CARE

Research commissioned by the Social Care Institute for Excellence (SCIE) and carried out by the National Centre for Independent Living (NCIL), Shaping Our Lives and the University of Leeds (2007) found that, although there are some positive examples of service user involvement in health and social care, experiences range from tokenism to true partnerships, with many current health and social care practices continuing to limit service user involvement. In particular, this research found that levels of involvement and participation vary across service user groups. There are some very positive examples of service user involvement in health and social care, such as Survivors Speak Out who have been vocal and involved in decision-making at both the individual and organisational level. Connexions is a public service that was introduced as part of the New Labour agenda to tackle social exclusion in young people (DH, 2003c) and offers support and advice to people between the ages of 13–19, primarily aimed at engaging young people with education, employment and training. The service is managed locally, and young people are actively involved in its design and delivery. However, there are also groups of service users whose voices are rarely heard and who continue to be marginalised, with minimal or absent involvement in the decision-making process.

Barriers to service user participation

- **Power** – unequal power relationships or perceptions about levels of power can limit service user involvement.

- **Differing priorities** – although there is a move towards personalisation and person-centred care, it has been argued that, in reality, health and social care professionals may continue to assess people for services and act as gatekeepers to public services. This means that rather than addressing service user needs and implementing a plan of care to address these needs, people are fitted into existing services, on the basis of a one-size-fits-all approach, which is counter to person-centred care (Parry-Jones and Soulsby, 2001).

- **Relationships between individuals and organisations** where equity was an issue have limited some service users' involvement in health and social care.

For example, in the report *Breaking the Circles of Fear*, the Sainsbury Centre for Mental Health (2002) found that many black people experienced poor quality services in mental health care, as stereotypical views, racism and a lack of cultural awareness contributed to poor assessment of needs, and subsequent treatments were dominated by interventions, including a heavily reliance on medication and restriction. This poor experience of care led to people being reluctant to seek treatment, which increased the likelihood of personal crisis and reinforced the stereotypical views of staff who perceived service users as potentially dangerous. The recommendations of the report are summarised as follows:

- ensure that black service users are treated with respect and that their voices are heard;
- deliver early intervention and early access to services to prevent escalation of crises;
- ensure that services are accessible, welcoming, relevant and well integrated with the community;

- increase understanding and effective communication on both sides including creating a culture which allows people to discuss race and mental health issues;
- deliver greater support and funding to services led by the black community.

These recommendations have been operationalised through various initiatives and policy directives achieving change through working with service users and gateway organisations. Good service user involvement encompasses engaging service users at every level of service provision, including education and training. Bennett and Race (2008) have demonstrated this through their work with service users in a higher education module for health and social care professionals. They discuss the way that they have approached inter-professional education and collaborative working in a module delivered to nurses and social workers. The module is delivered in partnership with a Young People's Group, which is involved at every stage of the planning and teaching of the module.

> The Young People's Group is involved in planning and delivering teaching throughout the module, with a clearly defined role in each of the six workshops. They provide a range of learning opportunities for students based on their own personal experiences and offer a unique perspective.
>
> (Bennett and Race, 2008: 223)

Case study

Shaping Our Lives is a user network that promotes collaborative working between service users and health and social care agencies:

- to support the development of local user involvement that aims to deliver better outcomes for service users
- to give a shared voice to user controlled organisations
- to facilitate service user involvement at a national level
- to work across all user groups in an equal and accessible manner
- to improve the quality of support people receive
- to enable groups to link to other user-controlled groups
- to develop links with world wide international user-controlled organisations.

www.shapingourlives.org.uk

Alongside the challenge to engage service users within a needs-led system of care delivery, there are also challenges to engage carers in the stages of the decision-making process. Walker and Dewar (2001) summarise satisfactory carer involvement in decision-making as follows:

- feeling that information has been shared with them;
- feeling included within the decision-making process (see Arnstein's Ladder of Empowerment on page 153);
- feeling that there is someone who can be contacted if the need arises – this is part of the preventative and early intervention priority outlined in *Shaping the Future of Care Together* (DH, 2009f) and is an important aspect of empowerment;
- feeling that the service is responsive to their needs – this can be related to the needs-led assessment and is an important aspect of assessment frameworks such as the Single Assessment Process; this can also be seen in policy developments, such as the Carers (Equal Opportunities) Act (DH, 2004b) (as discussed in Chapter 2).

Self-assessment

There has been a significant shift in the policy focus regarding the balance of power between service users and professionals in the last few years, with increased emphasis on service user involvement in decision-making at every stage of the assessment, planning, implementation and evaluation process. This creates a challenge in terms of new working practices and the professional role in engaging service users and carers in the cultural shift to person-centred care. Policy initiatives such as the *Expert Patient Programme* (DH, 2001a) (see Chapter 2) and the personalisation agenda (see Chapter 3) have placed the service user as expert in the decision-making process, leading to a greater emphasis on self-assessment and empowerment in the planning of interventions to address person-centred needs.

A simple definition of self-assessment is 'an assessment that is completed by the subject of the assessment without the immediate involvement of professionals, or a professionally-employed layperson' (Griffiths *et al.*, 2007:2). Self-assessment has been used in health and social care practice for some time, although it has become much more widespread within the modernisation agenda of the New Labour Government, as evidenced in various policies such as the *NSF for Older People* (DH, 2001c) and Single Assessment Process for Older People (see Chapter 3). The minimum expectations for self-assessment are summarised as follows:

- self-report – as distinct from examination and observation;
- self-completion – by the individual concerned rather than a professional, layperson or family member;
- self as the potential beneficiary of the assessment – as distinct from provision of a survey response for population needs assessment.

In addition, self-assessment can include one or more of the following:

- be self-initiated – rather than prompted by a professional;
- be self-interpreted – where the user is able to draw their own conclusions;
- be a prompt to self-care actions.

(Griffiths et al., 2007)

Parker and Bradley (2003) see self-assessment as a strengths-based approach to assessment, which reduces the power differential between the service user and health and social care practitioners, and recognises the service user as the expert in the assessment and management of their own care needs. The General Health Questionnaire is a good example of a self-assessment form, exploring people's subjective understanding of their health needs (available at **www.gp-training.net/protocol/docs/ ghq.doc**).

Self-assessment is central to person-centred care, independence and choice, but may also raise conflicts and challenges for health and social care professionals who have a role to safeguard vulnerable individuals as well as promote their choice and independence (see Chapter 3). Practitioners may have a difficult challenge in balancing the need for empowerment and enablement with the need to protect and safeguard, and may have to make complex decisions.

Case study

James, aged 23, is in the advanced stages of motor neurone disease, a disease that causes the progressive weakening of muscles. His mobility has dramatically deteriorated and he is now unable to walk at all. For some time, he has had progressive difficulty in using his arms and hands, and now finds even the simplest tasks difficult to perform. As his chest muscles have become affected, he suffers from severe shortness of breath on minimal exertion and has trouble eating and swallowing, as his tongue and other muscles around the mouth and throat have become increasingly weak. As a consequence, he has trouble swallowing saliva, resulting in dribbling from the mouth, which he needs help to wipe away due to the weakness in his arms and hands.

James knows that he is in the advanced stages of the disease and that he is approaching the end of life. He is mentally competent and has full capacity. You have been working with James for the last few weeks in the hospice where he is being cared for and have built up a good and trusting relationship. He has told you that he wishes to have a sexual experience before he dies, as he feels that he has not experienced this important aspect of adulthood, and asks if you would help him to find a prostitute who will help him to fulfil this need.

1. Think about how you would feel about such a request.
2. Although James is mentally competent and has capacity to make this decision, what risks might be involved for James?
3. What risks may need to be considered for others who might be affected by this decision?

This is a difficult scenario and raises a number of ethical and moral considerations. On the one hand, James has the right to make this decision as a competent adult who has the capacity to make autonomous decisions. However, on the other hand, the practitioner has to consider the impact of this decision not only on James but on other residents within the home, as well as reflecting on their own value base. Decision-making involves making judgements, where there is more than one answer to a particular issue. It involves thought on the part of the decision-maker and has an end product in terms of an action, which may include deciding to do nothing. In relation to the scenario above, decision-making also needs to be cognisant of our own personal values and impact on practice, our view about the nature and purpose of health and social care practice, as well as the influence of ethical theories in determining how we ought to behave as professionals. Information is also important in the decision-making process. In the scenario above, the practitioner would want to ensure that James had information about issues such as sexually-transmitted diseases, as well as the ability to make an informed decision based on the potential impact and outcomes of any decision.

Detmer *et al.* (2003) have argued that there is a need for much better provision of information to health and social care users in order to improve quality and efficiency outcomes of care. The following exercise identifies how the information a person has can impact on their decision-making and involvement in care.

Case study

The parents of a 20 month old baby girl know that she is allergic to eggs, and are worried about the severity of her reaction, which includes a facial rash and vomiting. Occasionally she reacts to other foods. The mother, worried about the reactions, talks to friends. One friend, who happens to be a nurse, suggests that she seeks help. The mother takes the toddler to her GP and asks for allergy testing. The GP is reluctant to refer her, suggesting that egg allergy is extremely common in babies and allergy testing is unpleasant for small children. The mother perseveres and is referred to a specialist clinic at the nearby teaching hospital.

At the referral, three months later, the toddler undergoes skin-prick tests for common allergens. Ten minutes later, the tests reveal that not only is she allergic to eggs but she is also allergic to nuts – an extremely serious allergy that is usually a lifelong condition. The doctor explains that the toddler must now totally avoid all nuts but, given that reactions to nuts have been mild, suggests that an adrenaline pen is not necessary.

Mother and toddler are ushered out to see the nurse. The clinic nurse, who is friendly and supportive, basically repeats the advice about the child not eating nuts or products containing nuts, and gives them a one-page information sheet and the name of an allergy support group.

The mother has access to the internet and looks up nut allergy on the search engine Google. The search turns up many different sites, including medical sites, patient group sites, food manufacturer pages, university dermatology departments, and more. Much of the information concerns the risk of an anaphylactic reaction, which can be fatal. The parents are very frightened by all this and are unsure how to apply it in their own case.

(Detmer *et al.*, 2003)

1. How well-informed are the parents?
2. What information do the parents need to help them to make decisions about the management of their daughter?

It can be seen from the case study above that there are numerous sources of information for the twenty-first century user of health and social care. We are experiencing a period of enormous change with the technological revolution and information and communication skills are increasingly important in providing people with information, as well as supporting independent living. Although rapid advances in technology pose a challenge for both users and practitioners in health and social care, self-assessment and independent living can also be facilitated through the effective use of technology.

SOCIAL INCLUSION AND EMPOWERMENT THROUGH INDEPENDENT LIVING – THE ROLE OF ASSISTIVE TECHNOLOGIES

Assistive technologies provide challenges in terms of a shift in ways of working but, at the same time, provide enormous opportunities for maximising people's independence and helping them to stay in their own homes or preferred place of care.

> Assistive Technology is any product or service designed to enable independence for disabled and older people.
>
> (DH, 2009j)

The principles of self-care and use of assistive technology are firmly embedded in government guidelines for care. In June 2008 the Department of Health published *Common Core Principles to Support Self Care: a guide to support implementation*, which was jointly developed by Skills for Health and Skills for Care. The key principles focus on supporting the modernisation and reform of services, with emphasis on user choice, control, independence and participation when using health and social care services. Support and enabling people to use technology to support their care and maximise independent living is enshrined in Principle 5 that:

> . . . requires workers to ensure appropriate equipment and devices are discussed, sources of supply are identified, and the use of technology is supported.
>
> (DH, 2009h)

Telecare

Telecare is a system of assistive technologies that offers an integrated approach to care within a personalisation framework and covers a wide range of technologies including falls monitoring equipment, smoke alarms, security alarms, etc. If telecare services are considered as an integral part of the assessment, planning and intervention process of care delivery, they can contribute to greater choice and control for individuals and maximise their independence.

Case study

Peter, aged 35, suffers from severe epilepsy and has always lived with his parents because of fears about the serious risks he would face if living on his own. However, having had an assessment of his needs for independent living, Peter has moved into his own flat. An epileptic monitoring system has been installed so that help can be alerted if he has a seizure and a smoke alarm has been installed in the kitchen in case he has a seizure when he is cooking. Peter is enjoying his independence and his parents feel reassured that he is supported and will receive the timely help that he needs if he has a seizure so that harm is minimised.

Telehealth

Telehealth can also provide benefits for service users and health and social care professionals alike, in terms of increasing people's choices over their preferred place of care, reducing inpatient stays and improving patient outcomes. Telehealth services can include home monitoring equipment that is linked to a central computer within a health care centre, so that the service user can be empowered to take control over their own health care monitoring, but also feel secure in the fact that they can communicate with health care workers if they have concerns. If we look at the case study of Frank on pages 19-20, we can see that Frank might benefit from telehealth to monitor his blood pressure and blood sugar, and so that he feels reassured that health care personnel are able to constantly monitor his health. This will also be beneficial in reducing his daughter's anxiety and is an efficient use of health care resources.

Information technology

Information technology can enhance people's sense of citizenship and social participation through opening up opportunities for interaction, through e.mail and other forms of online communication. It can also empower people to manage their own finances, shopping and other personal affairs rather than being dependent on others.

> ## Case study
>
> **Age Concern helps older people save online (04.09.08)**
> Saving money and finding good deals are a priority for increasing numbers of older people as the financial downturn deepens. In response to this demand, Age Concern's 'ITea and Biscuits' programme included guidance and training about online shopping during internet training and advice sessions.
>
> Online shopping has been shown to save people an average of £268 per year and price comparison sites allow people to research and make decisions within the comfort of their home. Online shopping also saves pensioners from having to carry goods home and already four in ten retired people are regular e-shoppers. Many older people ask specifically to learn about eBay and how it can help them generate cash and find bargains. Internet usage has overtaken gardening and DIY as a hobby for pensioners who spend an average of six hours a week online.

Silver Surfers is a group that was established to demonstrate the benefits of technology for supported living, increasing independence and providing greater choice and control and social capital for older people.

> The truth is that for older people, being online often makes more sense than it does for the young. Simple things such as online shopping can transform lives, while e.mail, messaging and chat can help maintain contact with friends and family all around the world.

The eighth annual Silver Surfers Day in the UK (2009) identified the benefits for older people of engaging with technology as shown opposite in Table 30.

Education and training for health and social care practitioners

These new challenges for practice can offer greater opportunities for independent living and control, but are also contingent upon having a health and social care workforce that is adequately educated and trained to work in collaboration with service users and carers, and to signpost appropriate services to meet their needs. Increasingly, the workforce

- If mobility is a problem, difficult or mobility-dependent tasks may be easier. For example, it may be easier to bank online rather than having to travel to a bank.

- The internet opens up opportunities for exploration of facts.

- The internet improves accessibility in that it is available 24 hours, every day of the year.

- It may be possible to maintain social relationships through the internet. Skype, for example, can help people to have 'face-to-face' conversations online. A project run by Digital Unite, called Schools for Silver Surfers, encourages school children to join up with people from sheltered housing and mentor them in technological skills. This not only develops important social relationships, but also helps to break down intergenerational barriers.

- It is possible to save money through using the internet to shop and pay bills. The Post Office estimates that savings of £840 per person can be made each year.

- The internet can help to equalise power relationships, as social variables such as age and disability are not readily apparent in internet communications.

- The internet can empower people and foster independence. The internet can help people to maintain the independence of communication and paying bills, rather than being dependent on other people to help them to do these things or to do them for them.

- If people are enabled to use the internet effectively, there are benefits in terms of self-esteem and self belief in the ability to master new tasks.

- There are health benefits in terms of self-help websites, but also the reduction of social isolation and depression.

- People's sense of personal value within an organisation or community is enhanced. For example, online voting can help to foster a sense of valued citizenship.

Table 30 The benefits of engaging with technology

involved in providing direct care is not professionally regulated and has not undertaken the education and training for professional practice that social workers and nurses have.

Braverman (1974) in his discussion of the manufacturing industry argued that work was organised within a hierarchical structure, with a division of labour and labour specificity. Tasks were broken down within the division of labour and there was a separation of mental and manual work, meaning that people at the top of the hierarchy would make the decisions about what needed to be done and would then delegate the tasks to those lower in the hierarchy, according to their levels of skills and experience. It could be argued that a similar division of mental and manual work is occurring within health and social care, with qualified practitioners carrying out the assessment and planning of care with service users and carers, but the implementation of that care often carried out by care assistants.

This raises challenges in terms of how the quality of care can be addressed, when the workforce may not have the same level of theoretical understanding about person-centred care. There are particular challenges in how care is delivered in an empowering and enabling way, rather than in a paternalistic way that disempowers people and creates dependency. This process needs to be monitored by professionals who are responsible for delegating caring responsibilities in the intervention phase of the ASPIRE process. Informed and managed delegation, alongside quality assurance mechanisms, must be used to ensure the quality of care delivered by all individuals involved in care is of the highest possible standard.

This raises challenges in terms of workforce development and the training, education, monitoring and regulation of service providers (including people paid as personal assistants within the personalisation and independent living agenda). In 2009 the Independent Safeguarding Authority was established to help prevent unsuitable people from working with vulnerable people. Under this scheme it is a criminal offence for those individuals who have been barred under the vetting scheme to apply to work with either vulnerable adults or children. However, how this will extend to the employment of personal assistants remains a contentious issue and questions have been raised about the safeguarding of vulnerable adults within the personalisation context. Health and social care professionals will need to be vigilant in their assessment and monitoring roles to ensure that vulnerability is not exacerbated by the new arrangements for social care.

The New Labour Government document *Putting People First* (DH, 2007b) set out its strategy for the development of the social care workforce:

> Our vision is one of a confident, enabled, and equipped social care workforce – a workforce who are able to deliver truly person centred care and understand and see the key role that they are making to delivering transformation. We see a workforce that is growing in confidence, learning and skills, led by inspiring leaders and championed by government. A workforce, which supports the cultural shift from:

- clients to citizens
- welfare to wellbeing
- expert to enabling
- transactional change to transformational change
- 'freedom from' to 'freedom to'
- safety net to spring board.

(DH, 2007b)

In future, social workers may have an important advocacy and brokerage role to support assessment and planning of work with service users, including those who are self-funding. This will require developments in education, regulation, practice and supervision to meet the challenges of these new ways of working as well as enhanced regulation, training and career structures for support workers (DH, 2007b).

Equally, with the vision for the future of nursing that has been set out in the document *Front Line Care – the report by the Prime Minister's Commission on the future of Nursing and Midwifery* (DH, 2010), it is recognised that truly compassionate care is 'skilled, competent, value-based care that respects individual dignity'. The delivery of such care requires the 'highest levels of skill and professionalism' and sees tackling poor practice as a major focus, with degree level education as a vital development, thus supporting the move to an all-graduate profession from 2013. The report goes on to describe a 'carequake' that is fast approaching – that is a massive and growing requirement to provide skilled care for people with many different needs – arising from long-term conditions, drug and alcohol addiction, the complex needs of ageing, problems in the early years, and much more.

Going on to question how health and social care services will deal with this demand in the coming decade the report (DH, 2010) states that there will need to be 'a much stronger focus on preventing and managing long-term mental and physical conditions, including the multiple, complex health needs associated with ageing' and advocates a stronger drive towards prevention and a more people-centred approach. It recognised the nurse's role as moving towards 'enabling, standing back and listening to what intervention is wanted by the person'.

CONCLUSION

The challenge for all those working in health and social care is how we can achieve the culture shift to enable and empower service users, and effectively use the ASPIRE process to address needs as defined by service users. The future role of health and social care practitioners will be to help service users to take control of their own lives and live as independently as possible. Although power has historically been concentrated in the hands of professionals within health and social care, this is changing and service users and carers often have different kinds of power resources that they can draw on to meet their needs. Good assessment of needs and planning and delivery of care will take account of these strengths and resources so that service users are not just empowered, but also emancipated to live in a way that addresses their needs.

Rights and entitlements are at the heart of government proposals for the future of health and social care and, although questions remain about how care will be funded in the future, there is a clear policy framework focused on prevention and early intervention, common processes of assessment, with collaborative working between professionals and with service users and carers, and a personalised approach to care, based on a fair system of funding.

> Users and carers are citizens. We expect to be respected as whole people and supported to achieve our aspirations. What needs to happen is that everyone recognizes us as the neighbour with the right to be included in society.
>
> (Scottish Executive, 2005)

Reflection	
Identify at least three things that you have learned from this chapter.	1. 2. 3.
How do you plan to use this knowledge within care practice?	1. 2. 3.
How will you evaluate the effectiveness of your plan?	1. 2. 3.

What further knowledge and evidence do you need?	1.
	2.
	3.

FURTHER READING

Leathard, A. and McLaren, S. (Eds) (2007) *Ethics: Contemporary Challenges in Health and Social Care*. Cambridge: Polity Press

This book examines theory, research, policy and practice in both health and social care fields. The importance of this approach is reflected in the growing emphasis on ethical issues in research and practice and, in Britain, on government policy aimed at improving partnership working across the two sectors. The analysis is set within the context of contemporary challenges facing health and social care, not only in Britain but internationally. Contributors from the UK, US and Australia consider: ethical issues in health and social care research and governance; inter-professional and user perspectives; ethics in relation to human rights, the law, finance, management and provision; key issues of relevance to vulnerable groups, such as children and young people, those with complex disabilities, older people and those with mental health problems; and lifecourse issues – ethical perspectives on a range of challenging areas from new technologies of reproduction to euthanasia.

Marquis, B. and Huston, C. (2008) *Leadership Roles and Management Functions in Nursing: Theory and Application*. London: Lippincott

Now in its sixth edition, this foremost leadership and management text incorporates application with theory and emphasises critical thinking, problem-solving, and decision-making. More than 225 case studies and learning exercises promote critical thinking and interactive discussion. Case studies cover a variety of settings, including acute care, ambulatory care, long-term care, and community health. The book addresses timely issues such as leadership development, staffing, delegation, ethics and law, organisational, political and personal power, management and technology, and more. Web links and learning exercises appear in each chapter.

Thompson, N. (2007) *Power and Empowerment*. Dorset: Russell House Publishing

This is a useful resource for exploring concepts of power and empowerment. It is accessible, explains complex concepts with clarity and provides points to consider, helping the learner to apply theoretical concepts to practice. There is a strong emphasis on social justice throughout the book.

Appendix 1

NHS	SAP Overview Assessment			
Contact and assessment details				

Contact and assessment details

Family name:			First Name:	Frank		
Preferred name:	Frank		Date of birth:			
NHS number:	XXX	Social care number:	XXX	Telephone:	XXX	
Assessor:			Role:			
Team/Ward:			Telephone:			
Assessment method:	☐ Telephone	☐ Face to face	Assessment location:			
Assessment date:		Other present:				

Brief description of person's presenting problems, difficulties or concerns

Type II Diabetes – 6 years.

Essential Hypertension

Lives alone

Feeling lethargic and tired

Poor nutrition

Unkempt appearance

Bereavement

Significant personal history *(include cultural/spiritual issues and/or personal preferences relevant to assessment)*

Married for 48 years. Wife died of cancer 2 years ago following 6 months of illness

Wanted to care for wife at home, but unable to achieve this due to complications prior to death

Lives alone

Daughter and son-in-law and 3 grandchildren 5 miles away

Son and daughter-in-Law and 2 grandchildren – some distance away but regular phone contact

Keen gardener

Wide circle of friends through British Legion Club

Formal care/support currently received *(frequency, nature of support, adequacy, etc.)*   ☐ None

Lifeline/Telecare	☐	Consultations with dietitian re control of diabetes
Nursing/Community matron	☒	3 monthly review of medication for essential hypertension by GP
Occupational therapy	☐	6 monthly review of hypertension by Practice Nurse
Physiotherapy	☐	
Dietetic	☒	
Podiatry	☐	
Medical care *(GP etc)*	☒	
Social care	☐	

Psychiatry/CPN/CMHN	☐
Speech and language	☐
Home care *(Council funded)*	☐
Day care	☐
Transport	☐
Homecare *(Private funded)*	☐
Meals on wheels	☐
Respite care	☐
Voluntary sector	☐
Other *(Specify)*	☐

| Name: | Frank | Date of Birth: | 74 years | Completed by: | |

Assessment Key: **Y** = Problem/need or yes; **N** = No need/problem or no; **?** = Possible problem; **N/A** = Not applicable; **N/K** = Not known; **U** = Unassessed

Sensory & communication

Eyesight	Y	Wears glasses for reading
Hearing	N	
Speech/Expression	N	
Understanding	N	
Other problem *(Specify)*		

Medical history *(recent admission in the last 28 days. Recent Procedures or falls in past year)*

Recent admission?	N	Main diagnosis: Diabetes
Recent procedure?	N	Additional Diagnosis: Essential Hypertension
Recent falls?	N	Other problem – Bereavement
Long term condition?	Y	
Main diagnosis?	Y	
Additional diagnosis?	Y	
Other problem *(Specify)*	Y	

Physical well-being

Physical well-being	Y	Lethargic and tired
Weight loss/gain	Y	Unkempt and withdrawn
Appetite/Diet	Y	
Allergies	N	Self reported loss of appetite and weight loss
Pain	N	
Skin (including pressure areas)	N	
Breathing	N	
Seizures/Epilepsy	N	Long toenails. Needs chiropody referral for foot care
General foot health	Y	
Swallowing	N	
Oral health status/Dental	Y	Wears dentures

Name:	Frank		Date of Birth:	74 years		Completed by:	
Bowels		N					
Continence (Urine)		N					
Continence (Faeces)		N					
Blood pressure		Y	Diagnosed with essential Hypertension (150/90) Prescribed 10 mgs Ramipril daily				
Temperature Pulse Respiration		N					
Other problem (Specify)							

Heath screening

Alcohol intake (units per week)		16 units per week		Smokes (number per day)	None (Quit smoking 30 years ago)
Routine screening	Y	Foot screens; retinal screens; kidney function tests. Cardiovascular risk			
Fluid intake	N				
Diet/intake	Y	Increased dependence on ready meals and take-aways associated with withdrawn status			
Vaccinations	N				
Exercise	Y	Exercise decreased as he has become more lethargic and withdrawn			
Alcohol use	Y	Self-reported drinking to cope with sense of loneliness			
Smoking	N				
Sexual Health	N/A				

Physical health needs identified? *If yes, consider further tests and/or referral e.g. for check-up*

Assessment Key: **Y** = Problem/need or yes; **N** = No need/problem or no; **?** = Possible problem; **N/A** = Not applicable; **N/K** = Not known; **U** = Unassessed

Psychological well-being

Reaction to bereavements/loss	Y	Still feels sorrow that wife died in hospital and feels guilty for not having been able to comply with her wishes to die at home
Depressed mood	Y	Seems depressed and withdrawn
Irritability	Y	Lethargic
Lowering of energy, drive and interest	Y	
Sleep	Y	Reports that he often wakes at 4am and cannot get back to sleep
Memory	Y	Sometimes forgets to take his medication
Orientation	N	
Anxiety/Phobias	N	
Indicators of Severe mental illness	N	
Risk behaviours	Y	
Substance misuse	N	Using alcohol to cope with loneliness
Self-neglect	Y	Social isolation

Name:	Frank		Date of Birth:	74 years	Completed by:	
Other Problem			Unkempt appearance. House smells fusty and damp.			

Does the person have a history of mental health problems?		☒ No	☐ Yes
Details:	Diagnosis *(if any)*:		

Mental health needs identified? *If yes, consider further assessment and/or referral.*

Medication

Current medications *(including non-prescribed, specify)*		☐ None reported		☐ Takes medication *(detail below)*
Ramipril 10 mg daily				

Ordering/collecting medications	N	
Taking medications as prescribed	Y	Sometimes forgets to take medication
Managing label/containers	Y	
Swallowing medicines	N	
Uses medication aids?	N/A	
Pharmacist support?	N/A	

Medication reviewed in past year? *(If no arrange GP review, if not known check with GP)*		☐ No	☒ Yes

Needs in relation to medication identified? *If Yes, make arrangements for review or appropriate referral.*

Assessment Key: **Y** = Problem/need or yes; **N** = No need/problem or no; **?** = Possible problem; **N/A** = Not applicable; **N/K** = Not known; **U** = Unassessed

Interpersonal relationships *(recent means the past year)*

Level of social contact	Y	Active member of British Legion Club until recently – lost some contact with his social network
Level of carer contact	Y	
Family/carer relationships	Y	Infrequent face-to-face contact with immediate family
Other relationships	Y	
Caring for others	N	Was an active member of the local church until recently and regularly provided flowers from his garden for the church displays
Child protection issues	N	

Name:	Frank		Date of Birth:	74 years	Completed by:	
Adult protection issues		N				
Recent victim of crime?		N				
Other problem (Specify)		N				

Social circumstances

Finances

Income and benefits	Y	Reliant on state pension and small war pension. May be eligible for additional benefits
Problems receiving benefits	N	
Finance Management	N/K	

Activities and employment

Problems to employment	N/A	
Access to employment	N/A	
Access to education	N/A	
Access to training	N/A	
Access to other activities	Y	
Access to services/amenities	Y	Always enjoyed gardening, but less involved in this in last couple of years

Housing situation

Location of housing	N	
Type of housing	N	
Security/type of tenure	N	
Access to home	N	
Access within home	N	

Home environment

Amenities	N	
Heating	Y	House feels very cold. Frank has a coal fire but rarely lights it, as he has nearly run out of coal. Hot water supply also affected by this
Existing adaptation	N	
Working smoke alarm	N	
General repair/condition	Y	

Name:	Frank		Date of Birth:	74 years		Completed by:	

Social needs identified? *If Yes, consider appropriate further assessments and/or referral*

Activities of daily living		Overall ADL score	

0 = Fully independent: NO assistance required from another person. May use equipment, adaptations, Telecare, etc. No need for support.	3 = Limited independence: ALWAYS requires supervision, prompting or assistance to undertake activity (other person needing to be present).
1 = Largely independent: OCCASIONAL reminder or prompting required; and/or difficulties in undertaking requiring OCCASIONAL help (include regular phone calls). Person not usually required to be present.	4 = High dependency: DOES NOT OR CANNOT undertake activity. Requires activity to be undertaken by ONE other person.
2 = Partial independence: OFTEN requires assistance, supervision or prompting (other person must be present). Can sometimes undertake independently.	5 = High dependency+: DOES NOT or CANNOT undertake activity. Requires TWO OR MORE people to undertake the activity.

Self-care		Frank capable of managing activities of daily living, but lethargy and apparent depression contributed to problems at present
Eating/Drinking	1	
Washing	1	
Bathing	1	
Toileting – day time	0	
Dressing/Undressing	0	
Grooming	1	
Everyday tasks		
Cooking/Food preparation	1	
Domestic tasks	1	
Shopping	1	
Mobility inside the home		
Moving	0	
Going up/down stairs	0	
Getting on/off chair	0	
Getting into/out of bed	0	
Turning in bed	0	
Lying to sitting	0	
Toileting – night time	0	
Mobility outside the home		No physical problems mobilising outside the home, but lacks motivation
Entering/leaving home	1	
Taking short walks	1	
Taking longer walks	1	
Using public transport	0	
Getting into/out of car	0	
Maximum level of assistance required?	☒ None	☐ 1 Person ☐ 2 People

Name:	Frank		Date of Birth:	74 years		Completed by:	

Does the person use aids, equipment or adaptations to support independence? *(detail if yes)*	☒ No	☐ Yes

Has a decline in skills been observed?	☒ No	☐ By person	☐ By carer	☐ By assessment/review

Can the person respond to emergencies?	☐ No	☒ Yes	☐ To a limited extent

Needs in ADL's identified? *If yes, consider OT assessment/referral and/or continuing care pre-screening*

Assessment Key: **Y** = Problem/need or yes; **N** = No need/problem or no; **?** = Possible problem; **N/A** = Not applicable; **N/K** = Not known; **U** = Unassessed

Family and carers		Notes
Presence of carer	N	
Carer's independence	N/A	
Carer's ability to cope	N/A	

Carers assessment	☐ Not discussed	☐ Declined	☐ Joint	☐ Separate

Assessment summary

Prior assessments and tests informing this assessment

Type	Date	Assessor	Role	Results and comments
Blood Pressure		Doctor/Practice Nurse		Maintained by Ramipril 10mg daily
Diabetes screening and assessment		Doctor Practice Nurse		On-going monitoring. Blood sugar levels maintained by diet
Lay assessment		Daughter		Reports that Frank is unkempt and withdrawn and has not been to the British Legion Club for some weeks

Name:	Frank	Date of Birth:	74 years	Completed by:	

Other contributions to this assessment *(via direct contribution or liaison. Who and what?)*

Risk arising *(assessor's view of risk – note differences with person/carer.)*　　　　**Risk score**

0 = No apparent risk. No history/warning signs indicative of risk.

1 = Some apparent risk (no previous history). No history indicative of risk but current factors/warning signs indicate possibility of risk.

2 = Some apparent risk (with previous history). History indicative of risk and current factors/warning signs suggest presence of risk.

Risk of falling	1	Tired and lethargic. Might be a risk of trip as house not being looked after properly
Risk re. physical condition	1	Concerns about diet and motivation to adhere to dietitian's guidelines
Domestic risk *(e.g. fire)*	0	Risk that self-care not being maintained adequately
Risk loss of autonomy	1	Stopped going to the British Legion. Not cooking
Risk to daily activities/routine	1	
Risk to relationships	1	Risk to relationships as he has stopped going to the British Legion and church
Risk of social isolation	1	
Risk of abuse/neglect by others	0	Unkempt and not looking after himself as well as he has done previously.
Risk of severe self-neglect	1	Daughter's concerns
Risk related to wandering	0	
Risk of suicide	1	Appears withdrawn. Waking early
Risk of deliberate self harm	1	Risk of neglect and excessive drinking
Risk of others from person	0	
Risk re. medication management	1	Sometimes forgets medication – risk of hypertension not being under control
Moving/manual handling risk	0	contributing to cardiac risk
Risk of pressure sores	0	
Risk of carer support	0	

Strengths and protective factors/Potential for self care *(e.g. personal qualities, social support)*

Frank has demonstrated independence and an ability to self-care until recently.

Good social networks, although some indication of isolation from these recently

Family support

Hobbies and interests

Spiritual network

Name:	Frank	Date of Birth:	74 years	Completed by:	

Summary of person's views/priorities

Keeping in contact with his family and other social support networks

Being able to contribute positively within his family and community networks (Frank does not want to feel that he is a burden)

Being able to heat the house effectively

Being able to sleep well

Summary of carer's views/priorities

Evidence of self-neglect

Concerns about Frank's ability to feed himself appropriately

Concerns about Frank's apparent depression and social isolation

Assessor's summary *(including overall impact of needs on person's independence, quality of life)*

Some evidence of self-neglect

Reduced quality of life due to increased social isolation

Compliance with medication regimes

Cold and damp house

Insomnia and early waking impacting on Frank's motivation and energy

Key needs identified	FACS Level (ASSD Only)
Compliance with medication	
Referral for investigation into possible medical cause of lethargy, withdrawal and insomnia	
Heating of house	
Social isolation and distance from social networks	
Ability to wash, dress and feed himself adequately	Low

FACS eligibility *(Adult social care)* ☐ None ☐ Low ☐ Moderate ☐ Substantial – low ☐ Substantial ☐ Critical

Name:	Frank		Date of Birth:	74 years		Completed by:	

Further actions

Has Direct Payments been discussed?		☒ No		☐ Yes but not required		☐ Yes and required

Continuing care indicated?	☒ No	☐ Yes	Telecare indicated?	☐ No	☐ Yes

Is the need for management of long term conditions indicated?		☐ No	☒ Yes

No further action	☐	
Information and advice	☒	
Ongoing monitoring	☒	
Referral(s) (indicate reasons)	☒	Chiropody for foot care. Referral for assessment of mental state due to lethargy, withdrawal and insomnia
Liaise with (indicate reasons)	☐	
Assessments (indicate reasons)	☐	
Care Plan/Carer support plan	☐	
Test/investigation	☐	
Intervention/Service provision	☐	
Carers assessment(s)	☐	
Other actions	☐	

I agree that the information in the form is correct and consent to the further actions identified.

Person signature	XXX	☒ Verbal Consent	Date	
Carer signature		☐ Verbal Consent	Date	
Assessor signature	XXX	☒ Electronic	Date	

Further notes/diagrams (using according to local protocol)

Appendix 2

A Nursing Care Plan for Frank

Date/Time	Potential Problem	Patient Goal	Nursing Intervention	Evaluation
	Frank appears withdrawn and reports feeling depressed. He has been neglecting his Activities of Daily Living (ADLs).	Assess and monitor his mood using the PHQ9. Longer term – engage with grief therapy. To engage with ADLs.	Refer to GP for assessment for anti-depressant therapy. Refer to Community Psychiatric Nurse for grief therapy. Help with sleep hygiene – set a routine for Frank to re-establish sleep pattern. Help Frank to attend to his ADLs – explain the importance of regular washing and grooming for self-esteem and personal hygiene.	
	Not eating regular meals. Unstable blood sugar.	To maintain blood sugar within normal parameters.	Refer to dietitian for advice on diet. Daily blood sugar recordings. Health education to teach Frank to monitor his own blood sugar. Refer Frank for the appropriate outpatient diabetic follow-up.	
	Cardiovascular risk due to hypertension.	To maintain blood pressure within normal parameters.	Help Frank to establish a regular physical activity routine. Discuss the use of telehealth to give Frank control over regular monitoring of blood pressure and blood sugar.	
	Frank is becoming increasing socially isolated.	Maintain existing social networks, prevent social isolation and establish new ones where necessary.	When Frank's mood has started to improve, facilitate Frank to re-establish contact with his friends and his previous other social contacts.	

Appendix 3

A Social Care Plan for Frank

Needs and Risks	Objectives	Services*	Outcomes
To keep warm and avoid the risk of hypothermia.	To ensure that Frank's home is properly insulated to avoid heat loss. To ensure that the heating is working properly.	Home Improvement agency to carry out repairs. Inform Frank about Age Concern Scheme for Approved Trades Persons. Arrange visit from Welfare Rights Officer to ensure that Frank is getting all the benefits he is entitled to.	Frank is warm in his own home and can afford to pay all his bills.
To have adequate nutrition to avoid risk of unstable diabetes.	To ensure that Frank has 3 nutritionally balanced meals a day.	Local lunch club. Mobile meals service. Friends from British Legion or church to visit Frank.	Frank maintains blood sugars in normal parameters and is maintaining weight.
To improve mental well-being.	To give Frank opportunities to talk about his feelings.	GP referral. CPN referral for grief therapy.	Frank feels more satisfied with his life. Frank is sleeping better.
Social contact to avoid risk of social isolation.	To enable Frank to enjoy other people's company. To re-establish existing social networks.	Friends from British Legion to visit Frank. Car sharing service to help Frank to get to church.	Frank's social contact has increased.
Increase activity to avoid social isolation and cardiovascular risks.	To enable Frank to enjoy his gardening. To help Frank feel that he is giving something to the community.	Local gardening club. Telephone advice from Age Concern.	Frank maintains his garden and begins to grow his own vegetables and flowers again. Frank contributes flowers to the local church and is able to share garden produce with family.
Some neglect in the home.	To enable Frank to feel safe and secure in his own home.	Inform Frank about Age Concern Scheme for Approved Trades Persons to check door and window locks. Fire Brigade to fit new smoke alarm.	Frank feels content and secure within his own home and feels more confident about cooking meals for himself.

References

Adams, R., Dominelli, L. and Payne, M. (2002) *Social Work: Themes, Issues and Critical Debates*. Buckingham: Open University Press

Allsop, J. (1984) *Health Policy and the National Health Service*. London: Longman

Andrews, H. and Roy, C. (1991) *The Adaptation Model*. Norwalk: Appleton & Lange

Annandale, E. (1998) *The Sociology of Health and Medicine: A Critical Introduction*. Cambridge: Polity Press

Arnstein, S.R. (1969) 'A ladder of citizen participation'. *Journal of the American Planning Association* 35(4) 216–224

Baldock, J., Manning, N. and Vickerstaff, S. (Eds) (2007) *Social Policy* (3rd Ed.) Oxford: Oxford University Press

Baldwin, N. and Walker, L. (2005) 'Assessment', in Adams, R., Dominelli, L. and Payne, M. *Social Work Futures: Crossing Boundaries, Transforming Practice*. London: Palgrave Macmillan

Banks, S. (2006) *Ethics and Values in Social Work* (3rd Ed.) Basingstoke: Palgrave Macmillan

Barclay Report (1980) *Social Workers: Their Role and Tasks*. National Institute for Social Work: Bedford Square Press

Barnes, C. (1991) *Disabled People in Britain and Discrimination*. London: Hurst

Beck, U. (1992) *Risk Society: Towards a New Modernity*. London: Sage

Benner, P. (1984) *From Novice to Expert*. California: Addison-Wesley

Bennett, A. and Race, T. (2008) 'Exploring young people's participation in interprofessional education, taking a children's rights approach'. *Learning in Health and Social Care* 7(4) 219–226

Beresford, P. (2007) 'Service users do not want care navigators'. *Community Care* 4.12.07

Bernstein, B. (1975) *Class, Codes and Control*. London: Routledge and Kegan Paul

Bilton, T., Bonnett, K., Jones, P., Stanworth, M., Sheard, K. and Webster, A. (2002) *Introductory Sociology* (4th Ed.). London and Basingstoke: Macmillan

Blair, T. (2003) *Fabian Society Annual Lecture – Progress and Justice in the 21st Century*. London: Fabian Society

Blaxter, M. (1990) *Health and Lifestyles*. London: Tavistock

Blaxter, M. and Patterson, E. (1982) *Mothers and Daughters: A Three Generational Study of Health Attitudes and Behaviour*. London: Heinemann

Bochel, H., Bochel, C., Page, R. and Sykes, R. (2005) *Social Policy: Issues and Developments*. London: Prentice Hall

Boud, D., Keough, R. and Walker, D. (1985) *Reflection: Turning experience into learning*. London: Kogan Page

Bradshaw, J. (1972) 'The concept of social need'. *New Society* 30. 640–3

Bradshaw, P.L. and Bradshaw, G. (2004) *Health Policy for Health Care Professionals*. London: Sage

Branfield, J. and Beresford, P. (2006) *Making User Involvement Work: Supporting Service User Networking and Knowledge*. York: Joseph Rowntree Foundation

Braverman, H. (1974) *Labor and Monopoly Capital: The Degradation of Work in the Twentieth Century*. New York: Monthly Review Press

Braye, S. and Preston-Shoot, M. (1995) *Empowering Practice in Social Care*. Buckingham: Open University Press

Brilowski, G.A. and Wendler, M.C. (2005) 'An evolutionary concept analysis of caring'. *Journal of Advanced Nursing* 50(6), 641–650

Bronfenbrenner, U. (1979) *The Ecology of Human Development: Experiments by Nature and Design*. Cambridge MA: Harvard University Press

Brophy, S., Snooks, H. and Griffiths, L. (2008) *Small-Scale Evaluation in Health: A Practical Guide*. London: Sage

Brotherton, G. and Parker, S. (2007) *Your Foundation in Health and Social Care*. London: Sage

Buchanan, R. and Carnwell, J. (2005) *Effective Practice in Health and Social Care – A Partnership Approach*. Buckingham: Open University Press

Burnard, P. (1994) *Effective Communication Skills for Health Professionals*. London: Chapman and Hall

Bury, M. (2005) *Health and Illness*. Cambridge: Polity

Businessballs (2009) PEST Market Analysis Tool. **www.businessballs.com/pestanalysisfreetemplate.htm** (last accessed 31.3.10)

Care Quality Commission (2008) Care Quality Commission Enforcement Policy Consultation **www.cqc.org.uk/pdf/CQC_enforcement_policy_consultation_08.pdf** (last accessed 02.02.09)

Care Quality Commission (2008a) About Us **www.cqc.org.uk/about_us.aspx** (last accessed 02.02.09)

Caris-Verhallen, W., Kerkstra, A. and Bensin, J. (1999) 'Non Verbal Communication in nurse–elderly patient communication'. *Journal of Advanced Nursing* 29(4), 808–18

Carper, B.A. (1978) 'Fundamental patterns of knowing in nursing'. *Advances in Nursing Science* 1978 1. 13–23

Cartwright, A. and O'Brien, M. (1976) 'Social Class Variations in Health Care', in Stacey, M. (Ed.) *The Sociology of the NHS*. Sociological Review Monograph 22, 1976. Keele: University of Keele

Cheal, D. (1988) *The Gift Economy*. London: Routledge

Close, L. (2009) 'Explaining about individual budgets and self-directed support'. *Working with Older People*. 13(2) 9–12

Commission for Social Care Inspection (2007) *Care matters: children's views on the government white paper*. CSCI: London

Coverdale, G. (2009) 'Public Health Nursing', in Thornbory, G. (2009) *Public Health Nursing*. Chichester: Wiley-Blackwell

Crawford, K. and Walker, J. (2008) *Social Work with Older People* (2nd Ed). Exeter: Learning Matters

Crinson, I. (2008) *Health Policy: A Critical Perspective*. Sage: London

Cross, T., Bazron, B., Dennis, K. and Isaacs, M. (1989) *Toward a Culturally Competent System of Care, Volume 1*. Washington, D.C.: Georgetown University

Dalrymple, J. and Burke, B. (2006) *Anti-Discriminatory Practice* (2nd Ed). Buckingham: Open University Press

Denney, D. (2005) *Risk and Society*. London: Sage

Department of Health (1983) Mental Health Act. London: HMSO

Department of Health (1989a) *Caring for People; Community care in the next decade and beyond*. London: HMSO

Department of Health (1989b) *Working for Patients*. London: HMSO

Department of Health (1989c) Children Act. London: HMSO

Department of Health (1990) National Health Service and Community Care Act. London: HMSO

Department of Health (1991) *Working Together*. London: HMSO

Department of Health (1993) The Allitt Inquiry. London: HMSO

Department of Health (1996) Community Care Direct Payments Act. London: HMSO

Department of Health (1997a) *The New NHS: Modern and Dependable*. London: HMSO

Department of Health (1998a) *Modernising Social Services: Promoting Independence, Improving Protection, Raising Standards Cm. 4169*. London: HMSO

Department of Health (1998b) *A First Class Service*. London: HMSO

Department of Health (2000a) *The NHS Plan*. London: HMSO

Department of Health (2000b) *The Cancer Plan*. London: HMSO

Department of Health (2000c) *The National Service Framework for Coronary Heart Disease*. London: HMSO

Department of Health (2000d) *Organisation with a Memory*. London: HMSO

Department of Health (2001a) *The Expert Patient: a new approach to chronic disease management for the 21st century*. London: Department of Health

Department of Health (2001b) *Valuing People: A New Strategy for Learning Disability for the 21st Century*, White Paper. London: Stationary Office

Department of Health (2001c) *The National Service Framework for Older People*. London: HMSO

Department of Health (2001d) *Seeking Consent: Working with Children*. London: HMSO

Department of Health (2001e) *The Essence of Care: Patient-Focused Benchmarking for Health Care Practitioners*. London: HMSO

Department of Health (2002) *Securing Our Future Health: Taking a Long-Term View – the Wanless Report*. London: HMSO

Department of Health (2002a) *Mental Health Policy Implementation Guide*. London: HMSO

Department of Health (2002b) *No Secrets: Guidance on Developing and Implementing Multi-Agency Policies and Procedures to Protect Vulnerable Adults from Abuse*. London: Department of Health

Department of Health (2002c) *Prescriptions Dispensed in the Community. Statistics 1991–2001 England*. London: HMSO

Department of Health (2002d) The Care Standards Act. London: HMSO

Department of Health (2002e) *The Single Assessment Process Guidance for Local Implementation*. London: HMSO

Department of Health (2002f) *Reforming Financial Flows: Payment by Results*. London: HMSO

Department of Health (2002g) *Requirements for Social Work Training*. London: HMSO

Department of Health (2002h) *Fair Access to Care Services*. London: HMSO

Department of Health and Home Office (2003) *The Victoria Climbié Inquiry: Report of an Inquiry by Lord Laming*. London: The Stationery Office

Department of Health (2003a) *Building on the best*. London: Stationary Office

Department of Health (2003b) *The National Service Framework for Diabetes*. HMSO: London

Department of Health (2003c) *Every Child Matters*. London: HMSO

Department of Health (2003d) *Fair Access to Care Services Guidance for eligibility criteria in adult social care*. London: Stationary Office

Department of Health (2004) *Addressing the Underlying Determinants of Ill Health*. London: Stationary Office

Department of Health (2004a) *Choosing Health*. London: Stationary Office

Department of Health (2004b) Carers (Equal Opportunities) Act. London: Stationary Office

Department of Health (2004c) Children Act. London: Stationary Office

Department of Health (2004d) *The NHS Improvement Plan*. London: Stationary Office

Department of Health (2004e) *Standards for Better Health*. London: Stationary Office

Department of Health (2004f) *House of Commons Health Committee: Elder Abuse: Second Report of Session 2003–4*, published 24 March 2004.

Department of Health (2005a) *Independence, Well Being and Choice*, Green Paper. London: Stationary Office

Department of Health (2005b) *National Service Framework for Long Term Conditions*. London, HMSO

Department of Health (2005c) Mental Capacity Act. London, HMSO

Department of Health (2005d) *Creating a Patient-led NHS: Delivering the NHS Improvement Plan*. London: HMSO

Department of Health (2006) *The Quality Standards for Health and Social Care*. London: HMSO

Department of Health (2006a) *Our Health, Our Care, Our Say*. London: Stationary Office

Department of Health (2006b) *Working Together to Safeguard Children*. London: Stationary Office

Department of Health (2006c) *Dignity in Care*. London: Stationary Office

Department of Health (2006d) *Essence of Care Benchmarks*. London: Stationary Office

Department of Health (2006e) *Action on Stigma: Promoting Mental Health, Ending Discrimination at Work*. London: HMSO

Department of Health (2007b) *Putting People First: a shared vision and commitment to the transformation of adult social care*. London: HMSO

Department of Health (2007c) *Children's Plan*. London: HMSO

Department of Health (2007d) Mental Health Act. London: Stationary Office

Department of Health (2007e) *Essence of Care Benchmarks*. London: Stationary Office

Department of Health (2008) *Health Inequalities; progress and next steps*. London: Stationary Office

Department of Health (2008a) *Care Programme Approach*. London: Stationary Office

Department of Health (2008b) *Personalisation Toolkit*. London: Stationary Office

Department of Health (2008c) *The Expert Patient Programme*. London: Stationary Office

Department of Health (2008d) *High Quality Care for All*. London: Stationary Office

Department of Health (2008e) Health and Social Care Act. London: Stationary Office

Department of Health (2009a) *Long Term Conditions* **www.dh.gov.uk/en/Healthcare/ Longtermconditions/index.htm** (last accessed 18.8.09)

Department of Health (2009b) *Carers Strategy*. London: Stationary Office

Department of Health (2009c) *Gold Standards Framework* **www.goldstandardsframework. nhs.uk/About_GSF** (last accessed 14.12.09)

Department of Health (2009d) *Common Assessment Framework for Adults*. London: HMSO

Department of Health (2009e) *The Laming Report*. London: HMSO

Department of Health (2009f) *Shaping the Future of Care Together*. London: HMSO

Department of Health (2009g) NHS ready for PROM Data **www.dh.gov.uk/en/News/ Recentstories/DH_094213** (downloaded 7.02.09)

Department of Health (2009h) *Research and Development Work Related to Assistive Technologies*. London: HMSO

Department of Health (2009i) *End of Life Care Strategy*. London: HMSO

Department of Health (2009j) *Research and Development Work Relating to Assistive Technology 2008–09*. London: HMSO

Department of Health (2010) *Front Line Care – the Report by the Prime Minister's Commission on the future of Nursing and Midwifery*. London: HMSO

Department for Children, Schools and Families and Department of Health (2009) *Social Work Task Force Final Report*. London: HMSO

Department of Health and the Department for Education and Employment (2000) *Common Assessment Framework for Children*. London: HMSO

Department of Health and Home Office (2000) *Framework for Assessment of Children in Need and Their Families*. London: HMSO

Department of Health and Social Services (1983) *Griffiths Inquiry Report*, cited in Crinson, 2008 (above)

Detmer, D.E., Singleton, P.D., MacLeod, A., Wait, S., Taylor, M. and Ridgwell, J. (2003) *The Informed Patient: Study Report*. Cambridge: Nuffield Trust

Dewey (1933) in Quinn (2000) *The Principles and Practice of Nurse Education* (4th Ed.). Cheltenham: Nelson Thornes

Dhalley, G. (1989) 'Professional Ideology and Organisational Tribalism? The Health Service-Social Work Divide', in Taylor, R. and Ford, J. (Eds) *Social Work and Health Care*. London: Jessica Kingsley

Dimond, B. (2005) *Legal Aspects of Nursing*. London: Longman

Dingwall, R. (1976) *Aspects of Illness*. London: Martin Robertson

Donabedian, A. (1966) in Al-Assaf, M.D. and Schmele, R.N. (1993) *The Text Book of Total Quality in Healthcare*. Florida: St Lucie Press

Donzelot, J. (1980) *The Policing of Families*. London: Hutchinson

Egan, G. (1990) *The Skilled Helper* (4th Ed.). Pacific Grove, CA: Brooks/Cole

Egan, G. (2002) *The Skilled Helper* (7th Ed.). Pacific Grove, CA: Brooks/Cole

Evers, A., Pijls, M. and Ungerson, C. (Eds) (1994) *Payments for Care: A Comparative Overview*. Aldershot: Avebury

Fawcett, B. and Karban, K. (2005) *Contemporary Mental Health: Theory, Policy and Practice*. London: Routledge

Featherstone, M. and Hepworth, M. (1991) 'The Mask of Ageing and the postmodern life course', in Featherstone, M., Hepworth, M. and Turner, B.S. (Eds) *The Body, Social Process and Cultural Theory*. London: Sage

Fernando (2001) in Richardson, J. (2009) 'Culture', in Glasper, A., McEwing, G. and Richardson, J. (Eds) *Foundation Studies for Caring*. Basingstoke: Palgrave Macmillan

Fischer, D.H. (1978) *Growing Old in America*. New York: Oxford University Press

Flanagan, J. (1954) 'The critical incident technique'. *Psychological Bulletin* 51, 327–358

Ford, P. and Walsh, M. (1994) *Nursing Rituals: Research and Rational Action*. Oxford: Butterworth-Heinemann

Forster, A., Lambley, R., Hardy, J., Young, J., Smith, J., Green, J. and Burns, E. (2009) *Rehabilitation for Older People in Long Term Care*. The Cochrane Collaboration. Chichester: John Wiley and Sons

Fredrikkson, L. and Lindstrom, U.A. (2002) 'Caring conversations – psychiatric patients' narratives about suffering'. *Journal of Advanced Nursing* 40(4), 396–404

Fruin, D. (2000) *New Directions for Independent Living: Inspection of Independent Living Arrangements for Younger Disabled People*. London: HMSO

General Health Questionnaire. Available at **www.gptraining.net/protocol/docs/ghq. doc** (last accessed 12.3.10)

General Social Care Council (2002) *Codes of Practice for Social Workers and Employers*. London: GSCC

General Social Care Council (2008a) *Fit for Purpose? The Social Work Degree in 2008*. London: GSCC

General Social Care Council (2009) *Raising Standards – Social Work Education in England 2007–8*. London: GSCC

Gibbs, G. (1988) *Learning by Doing: A Guide to Teaching and Learning Methods*. Oxford: Oxford Brooks University

Giddens, A. (1991) *Modernity and Self-identity: Self and Society in the Late Modern Age*. Cambridge: Polity

Giddens, A. (2006) *Sociology* (5th Ed.). Cambridge: Polity Press

Glasper, A. and Quiddington, J. (2009) 'Communication', in Glasper, A., McEwing, G. and Richardson, J. (Eds) *Foundation Studies for Caring*. Basingstoke: Palgrave Macmillan

Glennester, H. (1995) in Ackers, L. and Abbot, P. (1996) *Social Policy for Nurses and the Caring Professions*. Buckingham: Open University Press

Goddard, J. and Tavakoli, M. (2008) 'Efficiency and welfare implications of managed public sector hospital waiting lists'. *European Journal of Operational Research* 184 (2008) 778–792

Goldsmith, M. (2002) *Hearing the Voices of People with Dementia: Opportunities and Obstacles*. London: Jessica Kingsley Publishers

Graham, H. (1984) *Women, Health and the Family*. Hemel Hempstead: Wheatsheaf

Gramsci, A. (1971) *Selections from the Prison Notebooks*. London: New Left Books

Greener, I. (2004) 'Talking to health managers about change: heroes, villains and simplification'. *Journal of Health Organisation and Management* 18 (5) 321–335

Greenhalgh, T. (2000) *How to Read a Paper: The Basics of Evidence-based Medicine*. BMJ Books

Greenwood, J. (1998) 'The role of reflection in single and double loop learning'. *Journal of Advanced Nursing* 1998, 27, pp.1048–53

Griffiths, P., Ullman, R. and Harris, R. (2007) 'Self-assessment of health and social care needs by older people: Research Summary'. **www.sdo.lshtm.ac.uk** (last accessed 8.3.10)

Gubbay, J. (1997) 'Power: Concepts and Research', in Gubbay, J., Middleton, C. and Ballard, C. (Eds) *The Student's Companion to Sociology*. Oxford: Blackwell

Ham, C. (2009) *Health Policy in Britain (Public Policy and Politics)* (6th Ed.). London: Palgrave Macmillan

Hambridge, K. and McEwing, G. (2009) in Glasper, A., McEwing, G. and Richardson, J. (Eds) *Foundation Studies for Caring*. Basingstoke: Palgrave Macmillan

Hardey, M. (1998) *The Social Context of Health*. Buckingham: Open University Press

Hatton, K. (2008) *New Directions in Social Work Practice*. Exeter: Learning Matters

Hayes, S. and Llewellyn, A. (2008) *Fundamentals of Nursing Care: A Textbook for Students of Nursing and Social Care*. Exeter: Reflect Press

Hayward, J. (1975) *Information: A Prescription Against Pain*. RCN Research Series, London: RCN

Hazan, H. (2000) 'The Cultural Trap: The Language of Images', in Gubrium, J. and Holstein, J. (Eds) *Aging and Everyday Life*. Oxford: Blackwell

Healy, K. (2005) *Social Work Theories in Context: Creating Frameworks for Practice*. London: Palgrave Macmillan

Henderson, V. (1960) *Basic Principles of Nursing Care*. Geneva: International Council for Nurses

Henwood, M. (2008) 'The Principles of Personalisation Through Participation: Why Personalisation is here to Stay'. Implementing Personalised Care in Adult Services Conference. London, 2008

Heron, J. (2001) *Helping the Client* (5th Ed.). London: Sage

HMSO and Department of Health (1999) 'Supporting Doctors, Protecting Patients: A consultation paper.' HMSO, DH and the Sainsbury Centre for Mental Health

Hobsbawm, E. (1997) *The Age of Capital 1848–1875*. London: Abacus

Hockley, J. and Clarke, D. (2002) *Palliative Care for Older People in Care Homes*. Buckingham: Open University Press

Hogston, R. (2007) in Hogston, R. and Marjoram B.A. (Eds) *Foundations of Nursing Practice: Leading the Way*. Basingstoke: Palgrave Macmillan

Horner, N. (2009) *What is Social Work?* (3rd Ed.). Exeter: Learning Matters

Howe, D. (1992) *An Introduction to Social Work Theory: Making Sense in Practice*. Aldershot: Ashgate

Hudson, B. (2002) 'Interprofessionality in health and social care: the Achilles' heel of partnership'. *Journal of Interprofessional Care* 16(1) 7–17

Huycke, L. and All, A. (2000) 'Quality in health care and ethical principles'. *Journal of Advanced Nursing* 32(3) 562–571

Illich, I. (1976) *Limits to Medicine: The Expropriation of Health*. London: Marion Boyars

Information Commissioners Office (1998) The Data Protection Act. London: TSO

Iyer, P.W., Tapfich, P.J. and Bernocchi-Losey, D. (1986) *Nursing Process and Nursing Diagnosis*. Philadelphia: WB Saunders

Jasper, M. (1999) in Scholes, J., Webb, C., Gray, M., Endacott, R., Miller, C., Jasper, M.

and McMullan, M. (2004) 'Making portfolios work in practice'. *Journal of Advanced Nursing* 46(6), 595–603

Johns, C. (2004) *Becoming a Reflective Practitioner*. Oxford: Blackwell

Johnson, J. and De Souza, C. (2009) *Understanding Health and Social Care: An Introductory Reader*. London: Sage

Johnson, T. (1972) *Professions and Power*. London: Macmillan

Jones, D.P.H. (2003) *Communicating with Vulnerable Children: A Guide for Practitioners*. London: Royal College of Psychiatrists

Jones, H. (1994) *Health and Society in Twentieth-Century Britain*. Harlow: Longman

Kaplan, R. and Norton, D. (1996) *The Balanced Scorecard: Translating Strategy into Action*. Harvard: Harvard Business School Press

Kendall, J. (1992) 'Fighting back: Promoting emancipatory nursing actions'. *Advances in Nursing Science* 15(2) 1–15

Killick, J. and Allan, K. (2001) *Communication and the Care of People with Dementia*. Buckingham: Open University Press

King, R. and Raynes, N. (1968) 'An operational measure of inmate management in residential institutions'. *Journal of Social Sciences and Medicine* 2. 41–53

Kings Fund (2002) *Age Discrimination in Health and Social Care*. London: Kings Fund

Kitwood, T. (1993) 'Towards a theory of dementia care – the interpersonal process'. *Ageing and Society* 13(1) 51–67

Klein, R. (2005) *The Politics of the NHS* (2nd Ed.). Harlow: Longman

Kleinman, A. (1988) *The Illness Narratives: Suffering, Healing and the Human Condition*. New York: Basic Books

Lord Laming (2003) *The Victoria Climbié Inquiry*: Report of an Inquiry Presented to Parliament by the Secretary of State for Health and the Secretary of State for the Home Department by Command of Her Majesty January 2003.

Lord Mackay (1989) Hansard HL vol. 502, col. 488

Laybourn, K. (1995) *The Evolution of the British Welfare State*. Keele: Keele University Press

Law, M. (2000) 'Strategies For Implementing Evidence-Based Practice In Early Intervention'. *Infants and Young Children* Volume 13, Issue 2. pp. 32–40

Leece, J. (2004) 'Money talks, but what does it say? Direct payments and the commodification of care'. *Practice* 16(3) 211–221

Lee-Treweek, G. (1997) 'Women, resistance and care: an ethnographic study of nursing work'. *Work, Employment and Society* 11(1) 47–65

Lindberg, J.B., Love Hunter, M. and Kruszewski, A. (1990) *Introduction to Nursing: Concepts, Issues and Opportunities*. Philadelphia: Lippincott

Lindsay, T. (2009) *Social Work Intervention*. Exeter: Learning Matters

Llewellyn, A., Agu, L. and Mercer, D. (2008) *Sociology for Social Workers*. Cambridge: Polity

Llewellyn, A. and Hayes, S. (2008) *Fundamentals of Nursing Care: A Textbook for Students of Nursing and Health Care*. Exeter: Reflect Press

Llewellyn, A. and Mercer, D. (2008) 'Evaluation of Enablement Pilot Project in South Leeds for Leeds Social Services'. Unpublished Report

Lloyd, M. and Taylor, C. (1995) 'From Hollis to the Orange Book: developing a holistic model of social work assessment in the 1990s'. *British Journal of Social Work* 28(6) 863–878

Lockett (1997) in Hamer, S. and Collinson, G. (2001) *Achieving Evidence-Based Practice – a Handbook for Practitioners* (2nd Ed.). London: Elsevier

Lymbery, M. (2005) *Social Work with Older People: Context, Policy and Practice*. London: Sage

Lymbery, M. and Millward, A. (2000) 'The primary health care interface', in Bradley, G. and Manthorpe, J. (Eds) *Working on the Fault Line: Social Work and Health Services*. Birmingham: Venture Press/Social Work Research Association

Macionis, J. and Plummer, K. (2005) *Sociology: A Global Introduction* (3rd Ed.). Harlow: Prentice Hall

Marquis, B. and Huston, C. (2008) *Leadership Roles and Management Functions in Nursing: Theory and Application* (6th Ed.). USA: Lippincott Williams & Wilkins

Maslow, A. (1954) *Motivation and Personality*. New York: Harper

McClymont, M. (1999) 'Health and Wellness', in Heath, H. and Schofield, I. *Healthy Ageing: Nursing Older People*. London: Mosby

McDonald, C. (2006) *Challenging Social Work: The Context of Practice*. London: Palgrave Macmillan

McGinnis, E. (2009) 'Crisis Intervention', in Lindsay, T. (Ed.) *Social Work Intervention*. Exeter: Learning Matters

Means, R., Richards, S. and Smith, R. (2008) *Community Care: Policy and Practice (Public Policy and Politics)*. London: Palgrave

Mechanic, D. (1962) 'The concept of illness behaviour'. *Journal of Chronic Diseases* 15, 189–94

Meddings, F. and Haith-Cooper, M. (2008) 'Culture and communication in ethically appropriate care'. *Nursing Ethics* 15 (1), 52-61

Menzies, I.E.P. (1960) 'Nurses under stress: a social system functioning as a defence against anxiety'. *International Nursing Review* 1(6) 9–16

Midwinter, E. (1994) *The Development of Social Welfare in Britain*. Buckingham: Open University Press

Milner, J. and O'Byrne, P. (2009) *Assessment in Social Work* (3rd Ed.). London: Palgrave Macmillan

Moon, G. and Gillespie, R. (1995) *Society and Health: An Introduction to Social Science for Health Professionals*. London: Routledge

Moon, J. (2004) *A Handbook of Reflective and Experiential Learning: Theory and Practice*. London: Routledge

Muir Gray, J.A. (1997) *Evidence-based healthcare: how to make health policy and management decisions*. London: Churchill Livingstone

National Institute for Clinical Excellence (2002) *Principles for Best Practice in Clinical Audit*. Radcliffe Medical Press Ltd

National Institute for Health and Clinical Excellence (NICE) (2008) *About NICE*. **www.nice.org.uk/aboutnice/about_nice.jsp** (last accessed 7.2.09)

National Health Service Executive (1999) *Clinical Governance: Quality in the New NHS*. London: HMSO

Nettleton, S. (2006) *The Sociology of Health and Illness*. Cambridge: Polity

Neumann, M. (1995) *A Developing Discipline*. New York: National League for Nursing Press

Nursing and Midwifery Council (2004) *Standards of Proficiency for Pre-registration Nursing Education*. London: HMSO

Nursing and Midwifery Council (2007) *Essential Skills Clusters*. London: HMSO

Nursing and Midwifery Council (2008) *The Code: Standards of Conduct, Performance and Ethics for Nurses and Midwives.* London: HMSO

Nursing and Midwifery Council (2009) *Record Keeping Guidance for Nurses and Midwives* www.nmc-uk.org/aDisplayDocument.aspx?DocumentID=6269 (last accessed 18.9.09)

Office for National Statistics (2005) *Health and Social Care* www.statistics.gov.uk/cci/nugget.asp?id=1268 (last accessed 18.8.09)

Office for National Statistics (2008a) *Ageing – more pensioners than under-16's for first time ever.* www.statistics.gov.uk/cci/nugget.asp?ID=949 (last accessed 18.8.09)

Office for National Statistics (2008b) *Health & well being – living longer, more years in poor health.* www.statistics.gov.uk/cci/nugget.asp?id=2159 (last accessed 18.8.09)

Office for National Statistics (2009) *Expenditure on Health Care in the UK:* www.ons.gov.uk/about-statistics/ukcemga/publicationshome/publications/index.html (last accessed 24.08.09)

Oko, J. (2008) *Understanding and Using Theory in Social Work.* Exeter: Learning Matters

Oliviere, D., Hargreaves, R. and Monroe, B. (Eds) (1998) *Good Practice in Palliative Care.* Aldershot: Ashgate

Parker, J. (2007) 'The process of social work assessment, planning, intervention and review', in Lymbery, M. and Postle, K. (Eds) *Social Work: A Companion to Learning.* London: Sage

Parker, J. and Bradley, G. (2003) *Social Work Practice: Assessment, Planning, Implementation and Evaluation.* Exeter: Learning Matters

Parry-Jones, B. and Soulsby, J. (2001) 'Needs-led assessment: the challenges and the reality'. *Health and Social Care in the Community* 9(6) 414–428

Parsons, T. (1951) *The Social System.* London: Routledge and Kegan Paul

Patterson, E. (1998) 'The philosophy and physics of holistic health care: spiritual healing and a workable interpretation'. *Journal of Advanced Nursing* 27(2) 287–293

Payne, S. (2006) *The Health of Men and Women.* Cambridge: Polity

Pelling, M., Harrison, M. and Weindling, P. (1993) 'The Industrial Revolution 1750 to 1848', in Webster, C. (Ed.) *Caring for Health: History and Diversity.* Buckingham: Open University Press

Pearson, A. (Ed.) (1988) *Primary Nursing.* London: Chapman and Hall

Penhale, B. and Parker, J. (2008) *Working with Vulnerable Adults.* London: Routledge

Peplau, H.E. (1952) *Interpersonal Relations in Nursing.* New York: G. Putnum's Sons

Picker Institute (2009) *Using patient feedback – a practical guide.* www.pickereurope.org (last accessed 26.10.09)

Pollock, A. and Talbot-Smith, A. (2006) *The New NHS: A Guide to Its Funding, Organisation and Accountability.* London: Routledge

Punnett, R. (1994) *British Government and Politics* (6th Ed.). Aldershot: Dartmouth

Quilter, R.N., Wheeler, S. and Windt, J. (1993) *Telephone Triage: Theory Practice and Protocol Development.* New York: Delmar

Quinn, F.M. and Hughes, S. (2000) *The Principles and Practice of Nurse Education* (4th Ed.). Nelson Thornes: Cheltenham

Rapaport, J., Manthorpe, J., Moriarty, J., Hussein, S. and Collins, J. (2005) 'Advocacy and people with learning disabilities in the UK: How can local funders find value for money?' *Journal of Intellectual Disabilities* 9(94) 299–319

Reid, W. and Epstein, L. (1972) *Task-Centred Casework*. New York: Columbia University Press

Repper, J. and Perkins, R. (2003) *Social Inclusion and Recovery: A Model for Mental Health Practice*. Edinburgh: Bailliere Tindall

Rich, A. and Parker, D. L. (1995) 'Reflection and critical incident analysis: ethical and moral implications of their use in nursing and midwifery education'. *Journal of Advanced Nursing* 22. 1050–1057

Richardson, J. (2009) 'Culture', in Glasper, A., McEwing, G. and Richardson, J. (Eds) *Foundation Studies for Caring*. Basingstoke: Palgrave Macmillan

Rideout, E. (Ed.) (2001) *Transforming Nursing Education through Problem Based Learning*. London: Jones and Bartlett Publishers

Rivett, G. (2009) *National Health Service History* www.nhshistory.net

Rogers, L. (2009) in Glasper, A., McEwing, G. and Richardson, J. (Eds) *Foundation Studies for Caring*. Basingstoke: Palgrave Macmillan

Roper, N., Logan, W. and Tierney, A. (2000) *The Roper-Logan-Tierney Model of Nursing Based on Activities of Living*. Edinburgh: Churchill Livingstone

Routasalo, P. and Isola, A. (1998) 'Touching by skilled nurses in elderly care'. *Scandinavian Journal of Caring Sciences*, Volume 12, Number 3, pp. 170–178

Ryle, G. (1949) *The Concept of Mind*. London: Hutchinson's University Library

Sackett, D.L., Rosenburg, W.M., Gray, J.A., Haynes, R.B. and Richardson, W.S. (1996) 'Evidence based medicine: What it is and what it isn't'. *British Medical Journal* 312: 71–2.a

Sainsbury Centre for Mental Health, The (2002) *Breaking the Circles of Fear*. London

Salter, B. (1998) *The Politics of Change in the Health Service*. Basingstoke: Macmillan

Samuel, M. (2009) 'Direct payments, personal budgets and individual budgets'. *Community Care*, 8 April 2009 (available at www.communitycare.co.uk/articles (last accessed on 17.10.09)

Sartain, S.A., Clarke, C.L. and Heyman, R. (2000) 'Hearing the voices of children with chronic illness'. *Journal of Advanced Nursing* Oct 32(4) pp. 913–21

Schon, D. (1978) in Quinn (2000) *The Principles and Practice of Nurse Education* (4th Ed.). Cheltenham: Nelson Thornes

Scottish Executive (2005) *Changing Lives: Summary Report of the 21st Century Social Work Review*. Edinburgh

Shannon, C.E. and Weaver, W. (1949) *A Mathematical Model of Communication*. Urbana: University of Illinois Press

Shaping Our Lives. Available at www.shapingourlives.org.uk/about.html (last assessed 8.3.10)

Shu-Mei, Wu., Yu-Mei, Chao Yu., Cheng-Fang, Yang and Hui-Lian, Che. (2005) 'Decision-making tree for women considering hysterectomy'. *Journal of Advanced Nursing* Volume 51 Issue 4, pp. 361 – 368

Simon, A., Owen, C., Moss, P. and Cameron, C. (2003) 'Mapping the Care Workforce: Supporting Joined-Up Thinking. Secondary Analysis of the Labour Force Survey for Childcare and Social Work'. Research Report, Thomas Coran Research Unit, Institute of Education, University of London, April 2003

Smale, G. and Tuson, G. with Biehal, N. and Marsh, P. (1993) *Empowerment, Assessment, Care Management and the Skilled Worker*. London: HMSO

Social Care Institute for Excellence (2006) *Dignity in Care*. SCIE Briefing Paper 15.

Available at **www.scie.org.uk/publications/guides/guide15/index.asp** (last accessed 27.3.10)

Social Care Institute for Excellence (2007) *Developing Social Care: Service Users Driving Culture Change, Knowledge Review 17.* London: SCIE

Social Care Institute for Excellence (2008) *Dignity in Care.* SCIE Briefing Paper 15. Available at **www.scie.org.uk/publications/guides/guide15/index.asp** (last accessed 27.3.10)

Social Services Inspectorate (1997) *The Cornerstone of Care: Inspection of Care for Older People.* DH, London: HMSO

Stainton, T. and Boyce, S. (2004) '"I have got my life back": users' experiences of direct payments'. *Disability and Society* 19(5) 443–454

Stockwell, F. (1972) *The Unpopular Patient.* London: Royal College of Nursing

Stockdale, M. and Warelow, P. (2000) 'Is complexity of care a paradox?' *Journal of Advanced Nursing* 31(5), 1258–1264

Sutton, C. (1999) *Helping Families with Troubled Children: A Preventive Approach.* Chichester: Wiley

Swain, J., Finkelstein, V., French, S. and Oliver, M. (Eds) (1993) *Disabling Barriers, Enabling Environments.* London: Sage

Tanner, D. and Harris, J. (2008) *Working with Older People.* London: Routledge in association with Community Care

Thomas, D. and Woods, H. (2003) *Working with People with Learning Disabilities: Theory to Practice.* London: Jessica Kingsley Publishers

Thompson, N. (2005) *Understanding Social Work: Preparing for Practice* (2nd Ed.). Basingstoke: Palgrave Macmillan

Thompson, N. (2007) *Power and Empowerment.* Oxford: Russell House Publishers

Thompson, N. and Thompson, S. (2008) *The Social Work Companion.* London: Palgrave

Titterton, M. (2005) *Risk and Risk Taking in Health and Welfare.* London: Jessica Kingsley Publishers

Tones, K. and Green, J. (2004) *Health Promotion: Planning and Strategies.* London: Sage

Towle, A. and Godolphin, W. (1999) 'Framework for teaching and learning informed shared decision making'. *British Medical Journal* 18 September 1999; 319: 766–771

Tschudin, V. (2006) in Glasper, A. McEwing, G. and Richardson, J. (Eds) (2009) *Foundation Studies for Caring.* Palgrave Macmillan: Basingstoke

Tutton, E. (1991) 'Breaking the Mould' in McMahon, R. and Pearson, A. (Eds) *Nursing as Therapy.* Suffolk: Chapman and Hall

UKCC (1996) *Position Statement on Clinical Supervision for Nursing and Health Visiting.* London: UKCC

Ungerson, C. (1997) 'Social Politics and the Commodification of Care'. *Social Politics* 4: 362–381

United Kingdom Parliament (1998) Human Rights Act. London: HSMO

Walburg, J., Bevan, J., Wilderspin, J. and Lemmens, K. (2006) *Performance Management in Health Care.* London: Routledge

Walker, A. and Hennessy, C. (Eds) (2004) *Growing Older: Quality of Life in Older Age.* Buckingham: Open University Press

Walker, E. and Dewar, B. (2001) 'How do we facilitate carers' involvement in decision-making?' *Journal of Advanced Nursing* 34(3) 329–337

Wanless, D. (2004) *Securing good health for the whole population: final report.* Crown Copyright

Waterlow, J. (nd) *The Waterlow Scale* **www.judy-waterlow.co.uk** (last accessed 23.03.10)

Watson, J. (1985) *Nursing: Human Science and Human Care: A Theory of Nursing.* New York: National League for Nursing Press

Webb, A. and Wistow, G. (1982) *Whither State Welfare? Policy and Implementation in the Personal Social Services 1979–1980.* London: Royal Institute of Public Administration

Weber, M. (1976) *The Protestant Ethic and the Spirit of Capitalism.* London: Allen & Unwin

Webster, C. (Ed) (2001) *Caring for Health: History and Diversity* (3rd Ed.). Buckingham: Open University Press

White, K. (2002) *An Introduction to the Sociology of Health and Illness.* London: Sage

Whittington, C. (2003) *Learning for collaborative practice with other professions and agencies: A study to inform the development of the degree in social work.* London: Department of Health

Wilson, K., Ruch, G., Lymbery, M. and Cooper, A. (Eds) (2008) *Social Work: An Introduction to Contemporary Practice.* Harlow: Pearson

Winkleby, M., Feighery, E., Dunn, M., Kole, S., Ahn, D. and Killen, J. (2004) 'Effects of an Advocacy Intervention to Reduce Smoking Among Teenagers'. *Archive of Pediatric Adolescence Medicine* 2004; 158: 269–275

Woodman, T., Pee, B., Fry, H. and Davenport, E. (2002) 'Practice-Based Learning'. *European Journal of Dental Education* 2002; 6: 9–15

World Health Organisation (1984) *Report on the Working Group on Concepts and Principles of Health Promotion.* Copenhagen: WHO

Young, L. and Everitt, J. (2004) *Advocacy groups.* Vancouver, BC: UBC Press

Index

Lightning Source UK Ltd.
Milton Keynes UK
UKHW03f1534280618
324894UK00005B/234/P